Medical Masterclass

EDITOR-IN-CHIEF

John D. Firth DM FRCP
Consultant Physician and Nephrologist
Addenbrooke's Hospital
Cambridge

Scientific Background to Medicine 2

EDITORS

John D. Firth DM FRCP
Consultant Physician and Nephrologist
Addenbrooke's Hospital
Cambridge

D. John M. Reynolds MA BMBCh DPhil FRCP
Consultant General Physician and Clinical Pharmacologist
Department of Acute General Medicine
John Radcliffe Hospital
Headington
Oxford

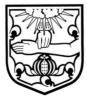

Royal College
of Physicians

Set and printed by Graphicraft Limited, Hong Kong

ISBN: 1-86016-216-9 (this book)
ISBN: 1-86016-210-X (set)

Distribution Information:
Jerwood Medical Education Resource Centre
Royal College of Physicians of London
11 St. Andrews Place
Regent's Park
London NW1 4LE
United Kingdom
Tel: 0044 (0)207 935 1174 ext 422/490
Fax: 0044 (0)207 486 6653
Email: merc@rcplondon.ac.uk
Web: http://www.rcplondon.ac.uk/

MEDICAL MASTERCLASS

Scientific Background to Medicine 2

Disclaimer

Although every effort has been made to ensure that drug doses and other information are presented accurately in this publication, the ultimate responsibility rests with the prescribing physician. Neither the publishers nor the authors can be held responsible for any consequences arising from the use of information contained herein. Any product mentioned in this publication should be used in accordance with the prescribing information prepared by the manufacturers.

The information presented in this publication reflects the opinions of its contributors and should not be taken to represent the policy and views of the Royal College of Physicians of London, unless this is specifically stated.

Every effort has been made by the contributors to contact holders of copyright to obtain permission to reproduce copyright material. However, if any have been inadvertently overlooked, the publisher will be pleased to make the necessary arrangements at the first opportunity.

Contents

List of contributors

Emma H. Baker PhD MRCP
Senior Lecturer and Honorary Consultant
St George's Hospital Medical School
London

John Danesh MBChB MSc DPhil
Research Fellow
Radcliffe Infirmary
Oxford

Stephen F. Haydock MA MB BChir PhD MRCP
Wellcome Research Fellow and Honorary Consultant Physician
Addenbrooke's Hospital
Cambridge

Aroon D. Hingorani MA MRCP PhD
Senior Lecturer and BHF Senior Fellow
Centre for Clinical Pharmacology
University College London
London

D. John M. Reynolds MA BMBCh DPhil FRCP
Consultant General Physician and Clinical Pharmacologist
Department of Acute General Medicine
John Radcliffe Hospital
Headington
Oxford

William Rosenberg MA MBBS DPhil FRCP
Southampton General Hospital
Southampton

Christopher J.M. Whitty MA MSc MRCP DTM&H
Lecturer and Honorary Consultant
London School of Hygiene and Tropical Medicine and
Hospital for Tropical Diseases
London

Foreword

Since its foundation in 1518, the Royal College of Physicians has engaged in a wide range of activities dedicated to its overall aim of upholding and improving standards of medical practice. *Medical Masterclass* is one of the most innovative and ambitious educational resources the College has developed, and while it continues the tradition of pioneering and supporting high quality medicine, it also makes use of modern day technology by offering computer-assisted learning.

The MRCP(UK) examination is crucial to the progress of physicians through their training. Preparation is not only essential for success in the examination, but it is also important for the acquisition of requisite knowledge, skills and attitudes appropriate for further training. With a pass rate of about 40% at each sitting of the written papers, the exam is a challenge. The College wishes to encourage excellence, and with this in mind has produced *Medical Masterclass*, a comprehensive distance-learning package designed to help candidates with the preparation that is key to making the grade.

Medical Masterclass has been produced by the RCP's Education Department. It represents a formidable amount of work by Dr John Firth and his team of authors and editors. I congratulate our colleagues for this superb educational product and wholeheartedly recommend it as an invaluable MRCP(UK) study aid.

Professor Carol M. Black CBE
President of the Royal College of Physicians

Preface

Medical Masterclass comprises twelve paper-based modules, two CD-ROMs and a companion website. Its aim is to help doctors in their first few years of training to improve their medical skills and knowledge.

The twelve paper-based modules are divided as follows: two cover the scientific background to medicine, one is devoted to general clinical issues, one to emergency medicine and practical procedures, and eight cover the range of medical specialities. Medicine is often fairly straightforward when the diagnosis is clear, but patients rarely come to their doctor and say 'I've got Hodgkin's disease': they have lumps. The core material of each of the clinical specialities is defined by case presentations in the first part of each module: how do you approach the man who has lumps? Structured concise notes on specific diseases follow later. All practising doctors know that medicine is much more than knowing lots of facts about diseases: how do you tell someone they've got cancer? How do you decide when to stop treatment? Most medical texts say little about these issues: *Medical Masterclass* does not avoid them, nor does it talk in vague and abstract terms.

The two CD-ROMs each contain 30 interactive cases requiring diagnosis and treatment. The format is remarkably close to real life: you see the patient and are told the story; you have to decide how to investigate and treat; but you can't see all the results before you start to make decisions!

The companion website, which will be regularly updated, includes self-assessment questions and mock MRCP(UK) exam papers. How much do you know, and are you improving? You will see how your score compares with your previous attempts, and also how your performance compares with others who have logged on to the site.

The *Medical Masterclass* is produced by the Education Department of the Royal College of Physicians. It has been specifically designed to support candidates studying for the MRCP(UK) Examination (All Parts). I have no doubt that someone putting effort into learning through the *Medical Masterclass* would be in a strong position to impress the examiners.

John Firth
Editor-in-Chief

Acknowledgements

Medical Masterclass has been produced by a team. The names of those who have written and edited material are clearly indicated elsewhere, but without the efforts of many other people *Medical Masterclass* would not exist at all. These include Professor Lesley Rees and Mrs Winnie Wade from the Education Department of the Royal College of Physicians of London, who initiated the project; Dr Mike Stein and Dr Andy Robinson from Medschool.com and Blackwell Science respectively, who have enthusiastically supported it from the beginning; and Ms Filipa Maia and Ms Katherine Bowker, who have run the office with splendid efficiency and induced authors and editors to perform to a schedule rarely achieved. I and the whole of the team of editors and authors are immensely grateful to all of these people for the energy that they have poured into *Medical Masterclass* in various ways.

John Firth
Editor-in-Chief

Key features

We have created a range of icon boxes to help you identify key information and to make learning easier and more enjoyable. Here is a brief explanation:

Clinical pointer
This icon highlights important information to be noted.

Further information
This icon indicates the source of further information and reference.

Hints
This icon highlights useful hints, tips and mnemonics.

Key points
This icon is used to highlight points of particular importance.

Quote
This icon indicates useful or interesting citations from notable individuals, including well-known physicians.

Think about
This icon indicates what the reader should reflect on after having read a passage from the text.

Warning/Hazard
This icon is used to indicate common or important drug interactions, pitfalls of practical procedures, or when to take symptoms or signs particularly seriously.

Statistics, Epidemiology, Clinical Trials, Meta-analyses and Evidence-based Medicine

AUTHOR (STATISTICS AND EPIDEMIOLOGY):
C.J.M. Whitty

AUTHOR (CLINICAL TRIALS AND META-ANALYSES):
J. Danesh

AUTHOR (EVIDENCE-BASED MEDICINE):
W. Rosenberg

EDITOR AND EDITOR-IN-CHIEF:
J.D. Firth

1 Statistics

Statistics is a large subject. Fortunately, physicians have to understand only a limited number of statistical techniques to conduct and understand the vast majority of clinical studies. All of these are simple and well worth mastering. The hard work will almost always be done by a computer; it is rather like driving—you don't have to know how a car works, but you do need to know how to steer it.

Continuous and categorical variables

Data are divided broadly into two categories:
- categorical variables are where the data fall into a few clearly defined categories, e.g. dead or alive, male or female, white, south Asian or Afro-Caribbean
- continuous variables are where the data can take on a whole range of values, e.g. age, blood pressure, temperature, blood glucose.

Continuous data can sometimes be turned into categorical data to make it easier to understand—we might, for example, categorize blood pressure into hypertensive or normotensive, or the blood glucose response as diabetic, glucose intolerant or normal. These divisions are often arbitrary, but we use them in clinical practice all the time.

Descriptive statistics

Continuous data

For statistical purposes continuous data have to be subdivided, as shown in Fig. 1, into:
- normal distribution
- skewed distribution.

This is far more important than is sometimes realized, because it defines how the data should be described, and tested, from then on. Central to this is the difference between the mean and the median. If a group of 251 students had their pulse taken, the mean is the sum of all the pulses, divided by the number of students (and may be a fraction, e.g. 76.6). The median is the pulse rate of the student who is the middle of the group if they are all lined up in order from the lowest to the highest (and will always be a whole number). In normally distributed data, the mean and median are about the same.

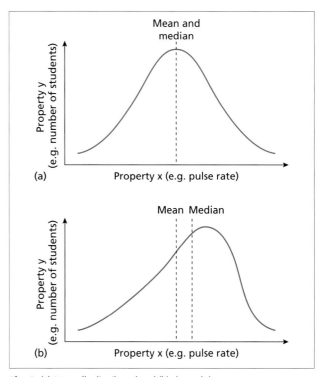

Fig. 1 (a) Normally distributed and (b) skewed data.

Normally distributed data

Normally distributed data are best summarized using the mean and standard deviation (e.g. a study will quote 'mean age 34.6, SD 5.6 years'). Statistical tests on normally distributed data also use the mean. The problem is that the mean will be wildly misleading if the data are highly skewed. If we did a study of alcohol intake sampling 100 medical students, the median alcohol intake might be 12 units per week, but a few keen members of a drinking club could easily push the mean up to 30 or more without affecting the median.

Seriously skewed data described by the mean may be misleading, and statistical tests using the mean will be uninterpretable.

Skewed data

Skewed data should always be summarized using the median, and statistical analysis requires different tests that use the median. The range is usually quoted (rather than the standard deviation, which is based on the mean), so, for example, 'median age 24, range 16–55'.

How do you decide whether data are skewed or not? Generally, the best way is to plot it out and look at it! But a reasonable rule of thumb is that data are skewed where the mean and median are more than slightly different.

Categorical data

Categorical data fall into neat blocks, and are usually summarized using percentages (e.g. 54% of the group were women, 46% were men).

Statistical tests of association

Most clinical studies are interested in whether there is a difference between one group and one or more others—e.g. comparing blood pressure in those with or those without a stroke, or whether drug A leads to fewer deaths than drug B. Statistical tests are therefore designed to find out whether the difference between one group and another may have arisen by chance alone. Formally they test the null hypothesis—which is that there is no difference between one group and another.

Once we have decided whether data are categorical or continuous and, if continuous, whether skewed or normally distributed, the correct statistical technique to use automatically follows. There is no magic to this. Table 1 compares the different methods of summarizing and testing categorical, normally distributed and skewed data.

Categorical variable against categorical variable

Say we wish to compare two groups of categorical data, e.g. dead/alive by drug/placebo. For looking at one categorical variable against another, the correct test is chi-squared (χ^2). Data are put into a 2×2 (or 2×3 or 2×4) table, and a chi statistic calculated.

There is a quick formula for calculating χ^2 for a 2×2 table. To calculate chi-squared for a 2×2 table, without a computer, consider the example of the effect of a drug on death in Table 2, where:

$$\chi^2 = n(ad - bc)^2/efgh.$$

Table 1 Describing and testing data.

Data type	Describe with	To test two groups
Categorical data	Percentage or proportion	Chi-squared (χ^2)
Normally distributed continuous	Mean and standard deviation	Student's t-test
Skewed continuous	Median and range	Wilcoxon rank-sum test/ Mann–Whitney U-test

Table 2 Effects of drugs A and B on patient death. Calculation of the χ^2 statistic for a 2×2 table: see the text for explanation.

	Drug A	Drug B	
Dead	a	b	$e\,(a + b)$
Alive	c	d	$f\,(c + d)$
	$g\,(a + c)$	$h\,(b + d)$	n (total)

The chi-squared statistic does not, in itself, mean anything concrete to the reader, but from it a p value is read off a statistical table (see below). For a 2×2 table, there are two degrees of freedom; for anything more leave it to the computer.

 Chi-squared (and its variations) is probably the single most widely used test in medicine, particularly in clinical trials, so it is worth being aware of a couple of pitfalls:
• if you construct your table and there are less than five in any one box, simple χ^2 is invalid, and you will need a variant called Fisher's exact test, which is slightly more rigorous
• if you have a zero in any box, seek statistical help, as χ^2 may not be valid at all.

Chi-squared can also be used to look for trends where there is a logical sequence of categories. You might be interested in the prevalence of angina in doctors you have divided into thin, medium and fat; there is a variation of χ^2 (χ^2 for trend) that can test for this. It is, however, easy to misuse, so seek statistical help.

Categorical variable against normally distributed continuous variable

For comparing a normally distributed continuous variable between two categorical groups, we almost invariably use Student's t-test.

Examples might be comparing blood pressure in a group on bendrofluazide and a group on captopril. The t-test calculates a statistic from which a p value is derived. The t-test is very robust, provided that the data are normally distributed. Tests on normally distributed data are also known as parametric tests.

Categorical variable against skewed continuous variable

When comparing data from two groups that are not normally distributed (skewed), we use non-parametric (also known as distribution free) tests. This will usually be the Wilcoxon rank-sum test (or Mann–Whitney U-test).

This is exceptionally laborious to do by hand, but easy for computers. It uses the median as its starting point. Again, a statistic is calculated, from which a p value is derived. As it is now just as easy to do non-parametric tests as parametric ones, it is reasonable to ask the question: why not do them in all cases? The reason is that the tests are less powerful, and therefore more likely to miss a true difference, so, provided that continuous data are normally distributed, the Student's t-test is preferable.

Continuous variable against continuous variable

In basic science, it may be necessary to compare one continuous variable against another (e.g. blood pressure against age), and this is usually done by one of a variety of regression methods.

The output is, however, often extremely difficult to summarize or interpret, even for those who have a firm grasp of the mathematics. It is worth knowing that these methods exist, but it is far better to reduce one variable to a categorical variable for studies meant to be interpreted by clinicians. Basing clinical decisions on the output of a regression analysis is usually difficult or impossible.

P values and confidence intervals

P values

All the tests quoted (χ^2, Student's t-test and Wilcoxon rank-sum) calculate a statistic from which a summary statistic, the p value, is derived. The p value is a measure of how likely a difference is to have arisen by chance alone.

However it is derived, the p value represents the same thing: the probability that an association could have arisen by chance. A p value of 0.5 means that there is a 50% chance that the difference is by chance alone, a p of 0.07 a 7% chance and so on. Traditionally, a p value of less than 0.05 (5% probability) has been taken as meaning it has not arisen by chance alone, but this is arbitrary.

p values

Two things must be clearly understood about a p value.
- The p value does not measure clinical or biological importance—it is not a direct measure of the importance of any effect and depends critically on the size of a study. A very large study or meta-analysis can generate very small p values for very small (and possibly clinically unimportant) differences, whereas a small study may fail to show an effect even if there is a large difference between one group and another.
- The more times one looks at the data, the smaller the p value that should be considered to be important—the conventional cut-off p value of 0.05 (a 1 in 20 probability of arising by chance alone) applies only if a single question is asked. If you test the data in lots of different ways (say 20 tests), or at many different time points, one of them will very possibly get a p value of less than 0.05 by chance alone. Statistical techniques are available to make explicit allowance for multiple testing of the same data (e.g. Bonferonni correction).

Confidence intervals

p values are a reasonable summary, but a more informative way of describing data and seeing how likely a difference is to have arisen by chance alone are confidence intervals. These are essentially doing the same thing as p values, but are even easier to understand, and with computers just as easy to calculate.

Formally, the 95% confidence intervals (95% CIs) around a value are the range within which there is a 95% chance that the true value lies. Similarly, the 95% CIs around a difference are the range in which there is a 95% chance that the true difference lies. The top value is the highest value it is likely to be; the bottom value is the lowest value. Confidence intervals can be quoted, but they can also be drawn (sometimes informally called 'error bars') on a graph, and this makes the concept much easier to understand (Fig. 2).

Assessing significant difference

P values and confidence intervals help to determine whether there is a statistically significant difference between two groups. They do not, however, provide a useful measure of how large or important that difference is. In clinical studies four measures are commonly used to do this:

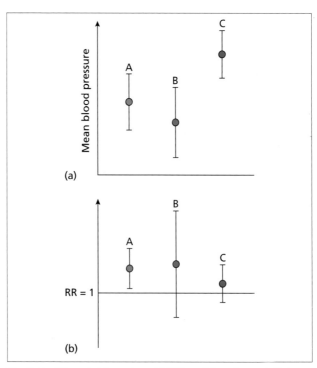

Fig. 2 Confidence level error bars: (a) 95% confidence intervals (CIs) around mean blood pressure in three groups. Where the CIs overlap, there will be no significant difference. C is significantly different from B, but not from A. (b) The 95% CIs around a relative risk (RR) for those given a new drug. Where they cross 1, there is no significant difference. Drug A has a significantly different effect. Drug B has a larger, but non-significant, effect.

1 The absolute risk reduction
2 The risk ratio
3 The odds ratio
4 The number needed to treat.

All of these measure the same thing, but express it in different ways. Most clinical studies comparing groups will quote one or more of these parameters, the 95% CI around the value of that parameter, with the p value testing whether any difference is statistically significant.

> Absolute risk reduction (or increase) = Risk in group 1 – Risk in group 2
> Risk ratio = Risk in group 1/Risk in group 2
> Odds ratio = Odds in group 1/Odds in group 2
> Number needed to treat = 1/Absolute risk reduction (or increase)

Consider the treatment of patients with myocardial infarction with aspirin. Let us define risk (of any outcome of interest, e.g. death) in those given aspirin (exposed) as $p1$ (probability 1) and risk in those not given aspirin (unexposed) as $p0$ (probability 0). Suppose in our example that the death rate is 9.4% in those given aspirin ($p1 = 0.094$) and 11.8% in those not given aspirin ($p0 = 0.118$).

Absolute risk reduction

The absolute risk reduction is the difference of outcome in one group compared with that in another:

Absolute risk reduction (or increase) $= p0 - p1$.

In our example, the absolute risk reduction produced by aspirin is $0.118 - 0.094$ or 0.024, meaning that, if 100 patients with myocardial infarction are given aspirin and 100 are not, then there are likely to be two or three more deaths in the 100 not receiving aspirin.

Risk ratio

The risk ratio or relative risk (RR) is simply the ratio of outcome in one group compared with that in another:

$RR = p1/p0$.

In our example, there is a relative risk of death after myocardial infarction of 0.094/0.118 or 0.80 if you take aspirin, meaning that those who took aspirin have 80% of the chance of dying compared with those who did not. Similarly, if you have a relative risk of 3.0 of developing skin cancer when you sunbathe, this means three times as many sunbathers develop skin cancer. As relative risks are a simple measure to understand, they are particularly appropriate for clinical trials. A relative risk of 1 means that there is no difference between two groups.

Odds ratio

Odds ratios (ORs) are not so intuitive, except to those who understand betting.

$OR = (p1/[1 - p1])/(p0/[1 - p0])$.

Taking our example again, the odds ratio of dying if given aspirin are (0.094/0.906)/(0.118/0.882) or 0.1038/0.1338 or 0.78.

As with relative risks, an odds ratio of 1 means that there is no difference between two groups, and the further we move away from 1 (up or down) the greater the difference. At small differences (as in our example), odds ratios and relative risks are roughly the same, but for big differences they become very dissimilar. A relative risk of 6 means that one group has six times the chance of having a particular outcome—an odds ratio of 6 represents a much smaller difference. The reason odds ratios are widely used despite being less intuitive is that they are easier to handle mathematically. Their danger is that people reading papers often think that a large odds ratio is the same as a relative risk, and they get an exaggerated sense of how big the difference is between one group and another.

The number needed to treat

The clinical significance of a reported reduction in absolute risk, relative risk or odds ratio is not always obvious. The concept of the number needed to treat (NNT) was devised to make this more obvious, enabling interpretation in terms of patients treated rather than the less intuitive probabilities.

$NNT = 1/Absolute risk reduction = 1/(p0 - p1)$.

In our example, the number needed to treat is 1/0.024 or 42, meaning that 42 patients with myocardial infarction must be treated with aspirin to prevent one death.

Sensitivity, specificity and usefulness of tests

Absolute risk reduction, the risk ratio, odds ratios and the number needed to treat are appropriate for looking at differences in risk between two groups, both for observational epidemiology and for clinical trials. In clinical practice, it is also necessary to have a statistical measure suitable for analysis of diagnostic tests.

Sensitivity

The sensitivity of a test is the ability of a test to pick up a condition:

$$Sensitivity = \frac{Number\ of\ true\ positives\ detected}{All\ true\ positives}.$$

A test that is 95% sensitive will detect 95% of all cases (or, put another way, miss 5% of cases).

Specificity

The specificity of a test is defined as follows:

$$\text{Specificity} = \frac{\text{Number of true negatives detected}}{\text{All true negatives}}.$$

A 75% specificity means that 75% of all true negatives will test negative, or conversely that 25% of true negatives will test positive.

Usefulness of tests

Sensitivity and specificity are absolute properties of a test, but do not necessarily demonstrate whether a test is useful in clinical practice. This depends just as much on the likelihood that a person has a condition in the first place. If the pre-test probability that a patient has a particular condition is very low, then most positive tests will be false positives, even if the test has, in absolute terms, a high specificity.

The practical usefulness of a test in a given population can be summarized using:
- the positive predictive value (the chance that a positive will be a true positive in that population)
- the negative predictive value (the chance that a negative will be a true negative in that population).

Positive and negative predictive values refer only to the population in which a study was done, because they depend as much on the prevalence of the condition that is being tested as on the accuracy of the test.

Power calculations and error types

Power calculations

It is essential that power calculations are performed before a study begins. A study that is underpowered is both pointless and unethical (see Section 3). The best years of many young researchers' lives have been wasted (along with a lot of money) pursuing studies that were clearly underpowered to detect the thing that they were looking for.

Physicians do not need to understand the mechanics of calculating power calculations; there are several formulae for different situations, and all statistical packages will do power calculations. The physician has to decide, however, on three things for a power calculation to be performed in a study comparing two groups:

1 How common is the condition in the reference population? Generally, the rarer the condition the larger the study will need to be.
2 How big a difference do you want to detect? The smaller the difference you want to detect, the larger the study will have to be.
3 How strict do you want to be in interpreting the data? There is a conventional default for this, but in certain circumstances you need to be stricter.

An example: let us say that you want to do a trial with expensive new drug A against conventional treatment in meningitis. Assuming that the two arms of your study are of equal size:
- If 30% die with conventional treatment and you were only interested in halving mortality (because smaller effects are not economically justifiable), you would need 266 patients.
- If 30% die currently and you were interested in detecting a 20% reduction in mortality, you would need 1782 patients.
- If 10% currently die and you wanted to halve it, you would need 948 patients.
- If 10% currently die and you wanted to detect a 20% reduction, you would need 6624 patients.

It is important to remember that power calculations are a minimum number.

Error types

Studies that are underpowered have the chance to fall into one of two major statistical errors:
- type 1
- type 2.

Type 1 error

A type 1 error is formally where 'the null hypothesis is falsely rejected'. In practice, this means that the study claims to find a difference that does not really exist, i.e. the result is just a statistical fluke.

The conventional cut-off for significance is p of 0.05, or a 1-in-20 chance. In theory, therefore, if 20 random small studies were conducted, you would expect to get one that was 'positive' by chance alone. The bigger the study, the less chance there is that this will happen. This is covered more fully under Section 3.

Type 2 error

A type 2 error is formally where 'the null hypothesis is falsely accepted'. This means that a researcher claims that there is no difference between two groups, when in reality the trial was just too small to detect a difference.

This is exceptionally common, even in papers published in the leading journals. To get a study capable of excluding a difference between one group and another, you usually need very large numbers (several thousands). Unfortunately, authors of papers often feel that a paper that claims to show 'drug A is as good as drug B' will be published, and one (however large and well conducted) that simply states 'we were unable to detect a difference between drug A and drug B, but the study was only capable of detecting a 20% difference' will not. Regrettably they are probably right; editors and readers like positive results (see Section 4).

Bland M. *An Introduction to Medical Statistics.* Oxford: Oxford University Press, 1987.
Kirkwood BR. *Essentials of Medical Statistics.* Oxford: Blackwell Science, 1988.

2 Epidemiology

Basic concepts

To understand clinical studies in the general medical press, it is essential to have a working knowledge of basic epidemiological methods, because most clinical studies and all clinical trials use these methods in both study design and analysis. There are only four basic classes of study design, although there are several variations on each theme, and it is important to decide which one a researcher is using. These are:

1 Cross-sectional studies
2 Comparative studies
3 Case–control studies
4 Cohort studies.

Each has advantages and limitations. To understand the pros and cons, it is helpful to remember a few simple concepts.

Exposure, outcome and association

All studies are looking at an exposure, and seeing whether it is associated with an outcome. This may involve:
• watching (an observational study)
• doing something (an intervention study).
The exposure might be a drug and the outcome a stroke (in a clinical trial), or the exposure might be radiation and the outcome cancer (an observational study). It must always be clear from the study design what exposure, or exposures, the study is investigating.

Epidemiology identifies associations between exposure and disease, but finding an association does not necessarily establish causality. There is, for example, an extremely strong association between having black skin and childhood malaria, yet nobody is going to claim that black skin causes malaria—it is just that most of those exposed to malaria are African. Associations have to be interpreted with caution and common sense but, if a very strong association is demonstrated (e.g. between lung cancer and smoking) and it makes biological sense, it is usually reasonable to assume that the exposure is a risk factor for the disease.

Prevalence and incidence

• Prevalence is the frequency of a condition in the community at a given point in time (e.g. 23% of the population aged over 85 have osteoarthritis).
• Incidence is the frequency of a disease occurring over a period in time (e.g. 1 in 1000 children had measles in the year 2000).

Prevalence is mainly useful for describing chronic conditions in which, once a patient has the condition, he or she has it for life. Incidence is almost always the best way to describe acute but short-lived conditions. The importance of this difference should be clear if we compare psoriasis and chickenpox.
• Chickenpox is a very common disease in the sense that almost everybody in the UK will have it once, but it is short-lived. At any given time, the prevalence of chickenpox is very low, but the incidence among children will be high.
• Psoriasis, on the other hand, is relatively much less common, but remains important for the rest of a patient's life. The number of new cases diagnosed in any given year is relatively small, so the incidence is small, yet the prevalence is relatively high, and gives a far better indication of how great a burden of disease there is in the community.

Sometimes it is obvious that it is best to use prevalence, sometimes incidence and sometimes both have advantages. If you want to study stroke prevention you will be interested in changes in stroke incidence, because it is the rate of new strokes that is important. If you are trying to plan the number of beds a health authority will need for stroke patients, the prevalence of those who have suffered a severe stroke will be more helpful.

Confounding

The last important concept is confounding, and this is the only thing in epidemiology that is not just applied common sense.

Confounding is a distortion where one exposure is associated with another exposure that is also a risk factor for a disease. This can cause incorrect conclusions to be drawn. It is important to remember that, to be a confounding factor, something must be associated both with exposure and with outcome. This can be expressed diagrammatically (Fig. 3).

It is easiest to understand confounding by considering an extreme example. If we are interested in risk factors for a disease, we might take a work sample where some of the men enjoy themselves down the pub in an evening, and another group go to the fitness club. We might ask the question: how protective is exercise for heart disease? If we look at the fitness enthusiasts, we would probably find that they have much less heart disease, and it would be tempting to claim that exercise is highly protective against heart disease—tempting but probably wrong.

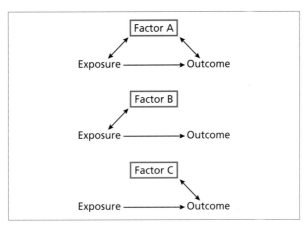

Fig. 3 Relationships between factors that do and do not confound a study. Only factor A is a confounding factor.

The groups who go to the pub and to the gym are likely to have a whole raft of different behaviours that are associated both with their pastimes and with heart disease. It is likely that the keep-fit enthusiasts will also eat lower-fat foods, drink less alcohol, smoke less and come from different socioeconomic backgrounds to those who go to the pub. On the other hand, there may be some people who started to go to the gym because they have heart disease. All of these will confuse the issue, because they are associated with both the exposure (exercise) and the outcome (heart disease), as seen with factor A in Fig. 3.

The art of epidemiology is to think about what might be confounding factors when you ask a question, which requires both imagination and general medical knowledge, and then to design studies that get around them, control for them or minimize them as much as possible.

2.1 Observational studies

Types of study

To identify associations and minimize confounding, four main epidemiological techniques have been designed. Each has strengths and weaknesses (summarized in Table 3). They are:
1 Geographical (ecological) studies
2 Cross-sectional (prevalence) studies
3 Case–control studies
4 Cohort studies.

Geographical studies (ecological studies)

Geographical studies are excellent at generating hypotheses, although less helpful at testing them. At their most basic, a physician sits in a library and notices from published data that, for instance, there is far more bowel cancer in

Table 3 Strengths (+) and weaknesses (–) of different observational study designs.

	Geographical	Cross-sectional	Case–control	Cohort
Rare disease	++++	–	+++++	–
Rare exposure	++	–	–	+++++
Multiple outcomes	+	++	–	+++++
Multiple exposures	++	++	++++	+++
Time relationships (incidence)	–	–	+	+++++

Britain than in Kenya. There are many possible reasons for this (genetic, sunlight, dietary—you think them up!). Some of these can be excluded because they are clearly daft, but this still leaves many possible exposures that could give rise to the disease. The genetic possibilities are most easily tested by looking at migrants—what happens to ethnic Kenyans who live a western lifestyle in Britain? If they take on the risk of a white resident, the risk factor is probably environmental; if they (and their children) keep the Kenyan risk, it is probably genetic. It may be both.

Medically important hypotheses that have been raised by geographical studies include some of the earlier evidence that hypertension plays a part in cardiovascular disease, that salt promotes hypertension, and that high-fibre diets are protective against colon cancer. Studies may sometimes simply use existing data to generate hypotheses.

Example 1: Geographical study

Figure 4 shows the correlation between the incidence of colon cancer in women and daily meat consumption per head of population in 23 countries [1].

The methodology used in geographical studies is very fast because the data are already gathered and in the public domain, but:
• it does not allow examination of any confounding factors
• 'routine' data (e.g. death certificates) are often inaccurate.

An alternative is to go out to do a survey in two areas. This is slower, but:
• data will be gathered in a standardized way
• information on confounding factors can be examined.

Example 2: Geographical study

A study of dental caries in children in six locations in the USA showed that the prevalence of teeth free of dental caries varied from 11% to 56%. All the worst three towns had a fluoride content in local water sources of less than 1.6 p.p.m.; all the best three had local fluoride contents of 1.7–2.5 p.p.m. This raised the possibility that fluoride in water protects against caries [2]. This was subsequently proved by an intervention study.

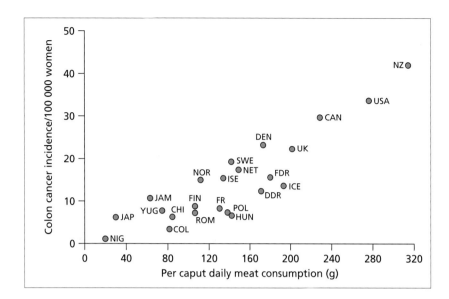

Fig. 4 Correlation between incidence of colon cancer in women and per caput daily meat consumption [1].

The main difficulty with geographical studies is that differences between two areas that cannot be controlled for cannot be excluded, nor can those that have not even been considered. Hypotheses generated by geographical studies therefore almost always need to be tested subsequently by other means.

Cross-sectional studies (prevalence studies)

Cross-sectional studies look at the number of cases of a disease at a particular point in time. The main advantage of cross-sectional studies is that they are excellent for estimating prevalence of a disease, and the methodology is simple. The main technical difficulty is ensuring a representative sample.

> **Example 3: Cross-sectional study**
>
> A sample of people aged 75 or over living in Cambridge in 1968 had a Mini-Mental State Examination and, if they scored less than 26 points, they were examined by a psychiatrist in a standardized way. The study demonstrated a 10% overall prevalence of dementia, with rates doubling every 5 years [3].

As cross-sectional studies are the best method of measuring prevalence of a condition, they are often used in public health for planning purposes. Cross-sectional studies can look at multiple possible outcomes (e.g. the same study could look for dementia and rheumatoid arthritis and diabetes) because the main problem is assembling the representative sample—once this is done, additional tests add little to the work.

In principle they can also look at multiple exposures. However, they are usually not good for testing hypotheses about the relationship between exposure and outcome in detail, because it is difficult to deal with potential confounding factors in a structured way. In addition, they are

not useful for investigating either rare diseases or rare exposures (a cross-sectional survey will not identify many, or any, examples), and they can look only at prevalence, not incidence, of diseases.

To get around these problems, two methods have been developed which are the backbone of almost all observational epidemiology:

- case–control studies
- cohort studies.

Case–control studies

In essence, case–control studies are simple. The researcher identifies cases of a disease and then selects a group of controls that do not have it, but are close to the patients who do in every other way. They compare the exposures of interest between the cases and the controls.

If the cases have higher levels of an exposure, it may be a risk factor for a disease. If the controls have a higher level of an exposure, it may be protective.

> **Example 4: Case–control study**
>
> Oestrogen pill use in 94 patients with endometrial carcinoma and 188 controls was compared. Of those with endometrial carcinoma, 57% took the pills compared with 15% of the controls. This raised the possibility that conjugated oestrogen may be a risk factor for endometrial cancer [4].

Case–controls have a number of major pitfalls, however, and can be done very badly indeed. The reasons almost always revolve around the selection of the controls. If the controls are badly selected, it may fatally bias the study. This is best seen with an example. Let us say that we wanted to study alcohol as a potential risk factor for breast cancer. We select our cases from the breast clinic, and take an alcohol history. Who can be the controls? The easiest thing is to select another group from within the hospital—orthopaedic wards are a favourite. The problem with this is that alcohol is a major risk factor for fracture, so the patients do not provide a good comparison. Similarly, those attending antenatal clinics (another traditional comparison for studies in women) are a bad comparison because pregnant women almost always cut down on alcohol. The chest clinic will usually contain smokers, and there is a strong correlation between alcohol use and smoking in many cultures. The gastroenterology wards are even worse. And so on.

There is nothing particularly clever about spotting these potential problems—it simply requires imagination, common sense and general medical knowledge. It is therefore surprising how many very poor control groups are published in the literature. There is no such thing as an ideal control group, but some are significantly worse than others. Generally the ideal is a community-based study, where the control lives in the same area as the case, but getting controls from the community is notoriously difficult and expensive.

With this caution, case–control studies are excellent in many situations and are the most widely used technique in observational epidemiology.

Pros are that, in general:
• they are quick and relatively cheap (you do it over a limited time period)
• it is possible to measure multiple exposures
• you can try to measure all potential confounding factors that you can think of
• they are excellent with rare diseases; as you start off with the cases, they can generally be as rare as you like, e.g. the amyloid clinic providing amyloid cases.

Cons are:
• the difficulty in selecting appropriate controls
• case–control studies are not good at looking at a rare exposure. Beryllium may be a serious risk for stomach ulcer, but as exposure to beryllium is so rare a case–control study comparing beryllium exposure in those with and those without an ulcer will probably not find it in either. This only ceases to be the case when the relationship between exposure and disease is so strong that almost all cases will have exposure (e.g. mesothelioma with asbestos).

Cohort studies

In cohort studies, one group with an exposure of interest is selected and another without that exposure. Both are then watched over time to see whether the group with the exposure develops the outcomes of interest more or less frequently. Clinical trials, which are discussed in much greater detail below, are a form of cohort study in which the researcher has set the exposure (e.g. drug or placebo).

Cohort studies have the same problem as case–control studies in trying to select two groups that do not auto-

Example 5: Cohort study

In 1951, 40 637 British doctors replied to a questionnaire about their smoking habits, and on the basis of this were classified as either smokers or non-smokers. They were sent subsequent questionnaires over a 10-year period to see if they were still smoking. All deaths and death register causes of death were notified to the study team by the office of the Registrar General. Death from lung cancer was linearly related to the amount smoked. Moreover, it was found that this increased risk dropped steadily after smokers gave up smoking, so that by about 15 years the excess risk had almost disappeared. This not only confirmed that smoking was detrimental, but that giving up smoking was beneficial. Data on the relationship of smoking to many other fatal diseases were also provided [1].

matically bias the result. Trials generally get round bias by randomization (see Section 3), but observational studies cannot. Take an example: is cotton dust a risk factor for asthma? The most obvious thing might be to compare workers in a cotton factory with a matched group from the same area. Unfortunately, this almost automatically biases the study, because employed workers are almost invariably healthier than the population as a whole for a variety of reasons, including pre-appointment health screening and the fact that the person with serious asthma may not be working at all (this is termed the 'healthy worker effect').

The pros of cohort studies are very considerable:
• You can usually define the exposure very closely.
• Multiple possible outcomes can be measured.
• They provide information not just on outcome, but on rate of outcome.
• Confounding factors can be measured in great detail prospectively, and do not generally suffer from the danger of recall bias.
• They are also particularly useful for looking at a rare exposure as a risk for common diseases, because the researcher predefines the exposure.

The cons of cohort studies are technical and practical:
• The main technical limitation is that they are not good for studying rare diseases or even moderately uncommon ones. You could study 700 men split into two exposure groups for 30 years, but would be unlikely to get a single case of hypopituitarism, or even hypothyroidism, in that time. Measuring differences of rates of these conditions in the two groups would therefore be meaningless, 0 : 0 being the likely outcome.
• The other main problem with cohort studies is that they take a long time and are therefore very expensive. There is often a high drop-out rate. In addition there is the very real possibility that, by the time you have finished the study, the burning question you set out to answer has been answered by other means, or that new techniques or definitions have rendered your initial question irrelevant or meaningless.

Nevertheless, observational cohort studies have provided many of the most robust insights in epidemiology.

Dealing with potential bias and confounding

Bias

Bias in a study is a flaw in design that leads to a built-in likelihood that the wrong result will (or may) be obtained. It cannot be controlled for or adjusted at the analysis stage.

The various examples given above under 'Types of study' show examples where bias may occur. If you read a paper that has clear, or potential, bias in the way that it is designed, it has to be considered uninterpretable. It might as well not have been done—in fact, in so far as it is misleading, it is better that it had not been done, because it is not only a great waste of time and money, but may also lead to dangerous mistakes. It cannot be stressed enough that bias is not a matter of faulty analysis but almost always of poor initial study design—a failure of common sense at the beginning of a study rather than of mathematics at the end.

Confounding

Confounding has to be taken into account in study design, but it is possible to make some adjustment for it at the analysis stage. There are two broad ways of dealing with confounding:
1 restriction
2 stratification.
These seldom eliminate confounding, but do reduce it.

An example: we might be interested in the extent to which smoking is a risk factor for heart disease among health-care workers. We know that men are at higher risk of heart disease than women. We also know that men smoke more than women. In addition there are several other factors that might well confound one another, including alcohol, stress, exercise, family history and socioeconomic background. We cannot eliminate these complex interactions, so we try to take them into account.

Restriction

One way to look at this problem is to try to restrict the analysis to people who are as similar as possible, e.g.

compare the smoking male doctors with the non-smoking male doctors, rather than considering all male health-care workers. This will remove a certain amount of the confounding, although not all. It will, however, make the results much less applicable, because they will say nothing about all other health-care workers or women.

Stratification

An alternative is to stratify. We compare the heart disease in smoking women with that in non-smoking women, and get a χ^2 for them. We repeat it for the smoking and non-smoking men, and get another χ^2 for them. We then combine the two χ^2 values, weighted by the relative number of men and women. This largely eliminates confounding by sex, because men are only compared with men and women with women. This method, called Mantel–Haenszel stratification, is a variation on the ordinary χ^2.

It is possible to stratify by several different confounding factors simultaneously, using more advanced statistical methods. The most commonly used is logistic regression. Provided that a study is large enough, this can control for many different factors simultaneously, so that, for example, young female teetotal smokers are compared only with young female teetotallers who do not smoke, while simultaneously comparing the male teetotallers with one another and the male drinkers with one another, and a grand summary statistic calculated for all of them together.

Mantel–Haenszel stratification can be done with a hand calculator; logistic regression can be done only by a computer, but for the operator it is equally easy because the computer takes the strain. Understanding how it is done is not necessary; physicians only have to understand that stratification can be done, and is relatively easy provided that potential confounding factors have been thought of and recorded for all cases in the first place.

1 Doll R, Bradford Hill A. Mortality in relation to smoking: 10 years observation of British doctors. *BMJ* 1964; i: 1399–410; 1460–7.
2 Dean HT. Endemic fluorosis and its relation to dental caries. *Public Health Rep* 1938; 53: 1443–52.
3 O'Connor DW, Politt PA, Hyde JB *et al.* The prevalence of dementia as measured by the Cambridge Mental Disorders of the Elderly Examination. *Acta Psychiatr Scand* 1989; 79: 190–8.
4 Zeil HK, Finkle WD. Increased risk of endometrial carcinoma among users of conjugated oestrogens. *N Engl J Med* 1975; 293: 1167–70.

3 Clinical trials and meta-analyses

Clinical trials are medical experiments. They are used to evaluate the potential benefits and the potential hazards of various medical 'interventions', including medicines, surgical procedures, diagnostic tests, management strategies and aspects of health policy. Meta-analyses of randomized trials are syntheses of studies about similar therapeutic questions.

Therapeutic versus preventive trials

• Therapeutic trials: these trials involve patients with existing disease. They try to determine the ability of an intervention to reduce symptoms, prevent recurrence, or decrease risk of death from that disease, e.g. can *Helicobacter pylori* eradication regimens relieve symptoms in infected patients with non-ulcer dyspepsia?

• Preventive trials: these trials involve evaluation of whether an agent or procedure reduces the risk of developing disease among those free from that condition at enrolment, e.g. can strategies of mass *H. pylori* eradication in the general population reduce the eventual incidence of gastric cancer?

The practice of medicine is increasingly based on clinical trials and meta-analyses of clinical trials, so physicians should be able to understand general issues related to their design, analysis and interpretation. The main focus of this section is on trials and meta-analyses with major clinical outcomes, such as death and serious morbidity.

Features of clinical trials with reliable methods

1 Design:
• proper randomization
• large number of events (deaths or serious morbidity)
• appropriate 'control' intervention (such as placebo tablets, standard treatment, different dosages of the same intervention).
2 Analysis:
• analysis by allocated treatments (i.e. an 'intention-to-treat' analysis)
• emphasis on the overall results (subgroup analyses can be misleading).
3 Interpretation:
• systematic meta-analysis of all the relevant randomized trials (emphasis on the results of one or another particular study can be misleading).

Large-scale randomized evidence

• Large treatment effects can usually be spotted in observational studies and in small trials
• Modest improvements in survival and in serious morbidity (e.g. reductions in the incidence of stroke or acute myocardial infarction) can still be medically important
• Large-scale randomized evidence is needed to confirm or exclude moderate effects.

Treatments with spectacular and unequivocal effects on death and major morbidity (such as therapies for malignant hypertension and diabetic ketoacidosis) generally do not require assessment in large clinical trials. Such effects can usually be spotted in observational studies (see Section 2) and in small trials, e.g. the benefits of *Helicobacter pylori* eradication in peptic ulceration are so striking that only a handful of small trials was needed to demonstrate them reliably (Table 4).

Large trials are needed to distinguish between treatments that are 'only' moderately effective and those that are ineffective. How small is a treatment benefit (or hazard) before it is worth knowing about? Reliable knowledge about changes in disease rates of even a few per cent can often be important. Applied to large groups of people, modest benefits from widely practicable treatments for common causes of premature death or serious disability can make big medical differences.

Demonstration of an important effect

Consider aspirin—the ability of daily medium-dose aspirin (75–325 mg) to prevent recurrences in a wide range of people with a previous history of myocardial infarction (MI) or occlusive stroke was reliably demonstrated by a meta-analysis of many randomized trials. Overall, about 9.5% (4835/51 144) of such patients allocated aspirin for a mean duration of about 2 years died or had a vascular event, versus 11.9% (6108/51 315) allocated control [1] (Table 5). Worldwide, there are more than 10 million deaths each year from MI and stroke, plus a comparable number of disabling non-fatal episodes. As aspirin is cheap, practicable and widely available, appropriately widespread use of it for the treatment and secondary prevention of vascular disease could well avoid more than 100 000 premature deaths annually.

Demonstration of no effect

Just as large-scale randomized evidence can demonstrate modest but important benefits that are overlooked in other trials, it can also refute claims of benefits made in smaller studies.

For example, infusion of magnesium salt in the treatment of acute MI was thought to reduce death by about a quarter. This practice was, however, based on studies involving only a few hundred deaths. The ISIS-4 randomized trial, by contrast, involved 58 050 patients with acute MI. About 7.6% (2216/29 011) of those allocated magnesium died within

Table 4 Randomized trials of *Helicobacter pylori* eradication strategies in peptic ulceration with about 1-year follow-up [10].

Abbreviated reference	Regimen / duration	No. of relapses[a]/total	
		Antibiotic arm	Control arm
Hentschel, *N Engl J Med* 1993; 328: 308	RMA/2 weeks	4/50 (8%)	42/49 (86%)
Graham, *Ann Intern Med* 1992; 116: 705	RBMT/2 weeks	6/47 (13%)	34/36 (94%)
Marshall, *Lancet* 1988; ii: 1437	BTi/8 weeks	5/20 (25%)	38/50 (76%)
Rauws, *Lancet* 1990; 335: 1233	BMA/4 weeks	3/24 (13%)	16/26 (62%)
Sung, *N Engl J Med* 1995; 332: 139	BMT/1 week	1/22 (5%)	12/23 (52%)
Graham, *Ann Intern Med* 1992; 116: 705	RBMT/2 weeks	2/15 (7%)	8/11 (73%)
Total		21/178 (12%)	150/195 (77%)

A, amoxycillin; B, bismuth; M, metronidazole; R, ranitidine; T, tetracycline; Ti, tinidazole.
[a]Refers to endoscopic ulcer recurrences.

Table 5 Summary of the overall results of trials of aspirin (or other antiplatelet drugs)[a] for the prevention of vascular events: the Antiplatelet Trialists' Collaboration (1994), involving a total of about 100 000 randomized patients in over 100 trials [20].

Type of patient	Average scheduled treatment duration (approximate no. of patients randomized)	Proportion who suffered a non-fatal stroke, non-fatal heart attack, or vascular death during trials		
		Antiplatelet (%)	Control (%)	Events avoided in these trials (per 1000)
High risk				
Suspected acute heart attack	1 month (20 000)	10	14	40 ($2P<0.00001$)
Previous history of heart attack	2 years (20 000)	13	17	40 ($2P<0.00001$)
Previous history of stroke or transient ischaemic attack	3 years (10 000)	18	22	40 ($2P<0.00001$)
Other vascular disease[b]	1 year (20 000)	7	9	20 ($2P<0.00001$)
Low risk				
Primary prevention in low-risk people	5 years (30 000)	4.4	4.8	4 ($2P>0.05$)

[a]The most widely tested regimen was medium-dose aspirin, involving a daily dose of 75–325 mg; no other antiplatelet regimen appeared significantly more or less effective than this in preventing such vascular events.
[b]For example, angina, peripheral vascular disease, arterial surgery, angioplasty, etc.

1 month, versus 7.2% (2103/29 039) allocated control [2]. This unpromising result suggested that the effect of magnesium had been overestimated by the earlier studies.

Reliable information generally comes from large randomized trials (and meta-analyses of such trials) that are interpreted cautiously.

Design of trials

Randomization

- Proper randomization should ensure unbiased comparisons
- Non-random methods involve biases that can mimic or obscure real treatment effects
- Randomization is the only method of allocation to achieve control for both known and unknown confounding factors.

Why should patients be allocated at random to different treatment strategies in clinical trials? The answer is simply because other methods are prone to confounding (see Section 2). Non-random methods (e.g. letting patients or doctors determine treatment allocation) are prone to biased assessments because the characteristics of patients allocated different treatments may differ in ways that could influence the results.

Methods of treatment allocation
1 Proper randomization (should avoid bias):
- computer-generated randomization
- random number tables.
2 Not proper randomization (prone to bias):
- assignment by odd/even number in the patient identification number, by date of birth, by date of presentation, etc.
- the patient or doctor chooses the treatment
- comparison with patients treated in the past.

Randomization ensures that each type of patient (e.g. young/old, male/female, low risk/high risk) should on average be allocated in similar proportions to the different treatment strategies.

The larger the trial, the more likely that randomization will produce perfectly balanced groups. This applies not only to characteristics that are measured routinely (e.g. age and severity of disease) but also to those potential confounders that may affect prognosis, but which may not be measured. Randomization is the only method of allocation to achieve control for both known and unknown confounding factors.

In a properly randomized trial, the decision to enter a patient is made irreversibly in ignorance of which trial treatments that patient will be allocated. Otherwise, foreknowledge of the next treatment allocation could affect the decision to enrol the patient, and those allocated one treatment might then differ in a systematic way from those allocated another. For example, if doctors determined treatment allocations in a clinical trial, people with more severe disease might preferentially receive the treatment believed to be more promising. As patients with more severe disease would be expected to have poorer outcomes than people with less severe disease, this method of allocation might obscure any treatment benefit.

Sample size

- A trial's relevant sample size depends on the number of clinical events (such as deaths and relapses) recorded after recruitment
- Without a few thousand events for analysis, moderate benefits or hazards of treatment on major outcomes can easily be missed
- Strategies to increase size include multicentre participation and studies of 'high-risk' groups.

The sensitivity of a trial depends not so much on the total number of people recruited into it but on the number of patients who die or suffer relevant clinical events before the statistical analysis takes place. Treatment differences can be detected in trials with varying numbers of relevant events. In general, to test reliably at least a 20% reduction in the primary outcome (such as death or recurrence of a cancer), a few thousand events are needed for analysis. Obviously, far more patients must be randomized to observe this number.

For example, in the ISIS-2 randomized trial of the treatment of acute MI, the 1-month survival advantage produced by aspirin was clearly demonstrated [3]. About 9.4% (804/8587) of the patients allocated aspirin died from vascular disease versus 11.8% (1016/8600) allocated to placebo control (Fig. 5). Nowadays, aspirin is routinely

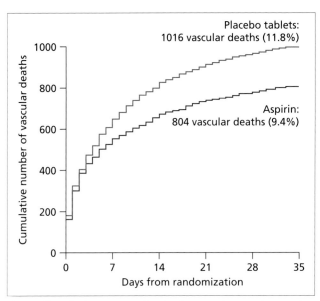

Fig. 5 Effect of administration of aspirin for 1 month on 35-day vascular mortality in the 1988 ISIS-2 trial, among over 17 000 acute myocardial infarction patients [3].

used in the emergency treatment of MI. Yet, if the ISIS-2 trial had been 10 times smaller (but still large in comparison with other cardiology trials at that time), it would not have been sufficiently sensitive, because 80 deaths in the aspirin group versus 100 in the placebo group would not have yielded a statistically significant result. Modest but important benefits (or hazards) cannot be confirmed or ruled out unless properly randomized trials have recorded sizeable numbers of events.

An obvious way of increasing a trial's relevant size is to increase the recruitment. This can be enhanced by:
- collaboration (such as the involvement of clinicians in many different hospitals)
- simplification of the study protocol (such as streamlining enrolment and follow-up procedures).

The ISIS-4 trial [2], for example, recruited 58 050 patients in only 20 months with the participation of clinicians in more than 1200 hospitals in 25 countries. Collaborators were asked to record only essential information and patients were then traced by national mortality statistics. There were 4319 deaths in these patients.

Other ways of increasing relevant size include prolonging the duration of follow-up and selecting high-risk populations to study, such as elderly people or those with previous disease. For example, the HOPE randomized study of ramipril versus placebo recruited people with a previous history of vascular disease or diabetes and monitored them for about 5 years [4]. This strategy yielded 1477 cardiovascular events—many more events than would have been expected in a briefer study or in a study of the general population. The HOPE study was able to demonstrate reliably that ramipril reduces death and vascular recurrences by about one-fifth. A later section of this module discusses yet another way of increasing the numbers of events available for analysis: meta-analysis of randomized studies.

The study intervention

- 'Factorial' studies assess several different treatments in the same trial
- 'Controlled' trials compare some intervention with a placebo, standard therapy or different dosages of the same treatment
- Poor treatment compliance by patients can mask real benefits.

'Factorial' trials

Most trials evaluate just one treatment, but this does not have to be so. 'Factorial' trials test two or more treatments simultaneously. Such comparisons can add to the scientific value and the practical efficiency of a trial ('two answers for the price of one').

For example, the ISIS-2 study was a factorial trial in which a comparison was made between placebo and each of two drugs, separately and in combination [3]. Patients with suspected MI were randomized to one of four treatments:

1 Intravenous streptokinase alone (1 500 000 IU over 1 hour)
2 Aspirin 160 mg daily alone
3 Both active drugs
4 Double placebo.

This trial not only showed that each of the drugs produced about a 25% reduction in mortality, but that they were additive in their effects (Figs 6 and 7). The ability to detect any 'interactions' between treatments is another advantage of factorial studies.

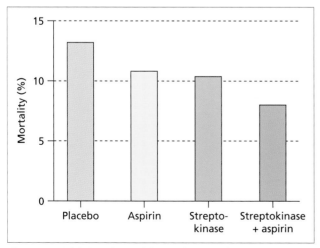

Fig. 6 Factorial design of ISIS-2 [3]. Mortality at 35 days: both streptokinase and aspirin produced a >20% reduction in mortality, and the effect of the two therapies was additive.

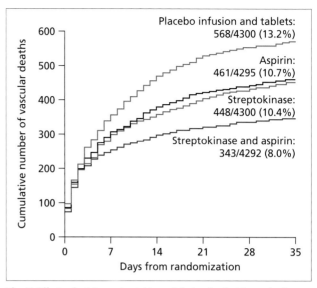

Fig. 7 Effects of a 1-hour streptokinase infusion (and of 1 month of aspirin) on 35-day vascular mortality in ISIS-2 [3].

'Controlled' trials

'Controlled' trials refer to studies in which the effects of a new 'test' treatment are compared with those of an existing therapy—either inactive (placebo) or active. If there is already a treatment of proven value, patients in the control arm should receive it.

For example, the SEARCH randomized study is comparing 80 mg simvastatin daily versus 20 mg simvastatin in 12 000 patients with a previous history of MI. The trial's control treatment is such because the 4S trial previously demonstrated that 20 mg simvastatin produces about a 33% reduction in death and recurrences in such patients compared with placebo [5].

If a standard treatment does not exist, placebo control may help to avoid biases that might arise through knowledge of a patient's treatment status (in 'double-blind' studies treatment status is concealed from both patients and doctors). Such measures are particularly necessary when there is a substantial degree of subjectivity, such as the self-reporting of symptoms in trials of non-ulcer dyspepsia and *H. pylori* eradication.

Compliance

There are many reasons why patients fail to take their medications in clinical trials (or in routine clinical practice): they forget, develop side effects, withdraw consent, obtain alternative treatments on their own initiative, etc. Whatever the reasons for it, imperfect compliance has the same effect: it decreases the ability of a trial to detect differences between treatments.

Non-compliance is a particular example of a more general problem in trials—ensuring that experimental contrast between treatment and control groups persists for the whole duration of the study. A suboptimal therapy can blunt or obscure real treatment benefits (such as *H. pylori* eradication regimens with low bacterial 'kill rates'). A treatment with an unsustained action has the same effect (such as re-infection with *H. pylori* after successful eradication).

Overlap between treatment groups is particularly likely in studies of behavioural interventions. For example, in the MRFIT randomized study, 12 866 men at high risk of coronary heart disease received either a special programme to reduce coronary risk factors (such as smoking, blood pressure and blood cholesterol) or usual care [6]. By the end of the study, risk factors in the two groups were more similar than anticipated, partly because some men allocated special treatment did not comply with it, and partly because men allocated usual care adopted healthier habits by the end of the study. Perhaps as a consequence, the study did not demonstrate conclusive benefits for cardiac mortality.

Analysis of trials

Stopping a trial prematurely

Trials stopped prematurely are prone to exaggeration.

A trial may be stopped before its scheduled duration if clear evidence of a benefit or a hazard emerges in the interim. A data monitoring committee, independent of the study investigators, usually monitors interim results. The goal is to protect the interests of the participants in the study as well as the larger population of future potential patients.

This can be a tricky balance to strike. For example, a randomized study compared extracorporeal membrane oxygenation with standard medical treatment in newborns with persistent pulmonary hypertension [7]. It was stopped prematurely when four of the ten infants allocated standard treatment died, compared with none of the nine allocated extracorporeal membrane oxygenation. These numbers were small, and many clinicians considered the results unconvincing. A much larger trial, reported several years after the original study, provided much more reliable evidence of a benefit, and this evidence persuaded many more clinicians to adopt extracorporeal membrane oxygenation treatment [8]. During this period of uncertainty, lack of convincing evidence may well have led to fewer newborns worldwide receiving the new treatment than would have been the case had the original trial continued longer.

Scepticism about interim findings is usually justified.

Experience has shown that emerging trends based on small numbers might well be transient and disappear, or

even reverse, after data have accumulated from a larger sample. For example, three separate interim analyses during the first 30 months of the Coronary Drug Project randomized study suggested fewer deaths in those allocated clofibrate than in those allocated placebo ($P <0.05$) [9]. The data monitoring committee, however, appropriately regarded this evidence as too weak to warrant stopping early. When the final results were analysed 3 years later, deaths in the clofibrate group were nearly identical to those of the placebo group (25.5% vs 25.4%).

'Intention-to-treat' analysis

The main comparison in a trial should be an 'intention-to-treat' analysis, i.e. comparison of outcomes among all those originally allocated one treatment with all those allocated the other treatment.

It is easy to spoil the benefits of random allocation by an inappropriate analysis of data. A common but mistaken practice is to exclude randomized patients from the main analysis, usually because they were either non-compliant with the study treatment or lost to follow-up. This approach can distort results if the prognosis of those excluded from one treatment group differs from the prognosis of those excluded from the other group.

Such confounding was demonstrated by the investigators in the Coronary Drug Project trial. Patients who took at least 80% of their allocated clofibrate had substantially lower 5-year mortality rates than those who did not (15.0% vs 24.6%, respectively), but there was an even larger difference in mortality between good and poor compliers in the placebo group (15.1% vs 28.3%, respectively) [9].

The main statistical analysis in any trial should compare outcome among all patients originally allocated one treatment (even though some of them may not have actually received it) with outcome among all those allocated the other treatment. Nowadays, leading medical journals require the reporting of such 'intention-to-treat' analyses for randomized trials, but this does not guarantee that they are actually done. For example, four randomized trials of *H. pylori* eradication in non-ulcer dyspepsia, all published in leading journals between 1998 and 2000, stated policies of intention-to-treat analyses. Each, however, excluded certain randomized patients, representing 6% of the total randomized in the four trials combined [10].

Exploratory analyses and subgroups

• Trust an overall result of a study much more than subdivisions of data
• Subgroup analyses can be seriously misleading.

A subgroup analysis refers to subdivision of the main comparison in a study. As patients can be grouped by many different characteristics (age, sex, severity of disease, etc.) and by many combinations of characteristics (young men with severe disease, old women with minor disease, etc.), exploratory analyses of subgroups can be numerous.

This is a problem because each additional statistical comparison increases the risk of a false-positive result, particularly when sparse data are finely divided. Subgroup analyses can either produce spurious results ('torture the data enough, and eventually it will confess') or overlook real differences between subgroups. Only certain very large studies (or certain large meta-analyses—see later) have adequate precision to make reliable comparisons about possible treatment differences in subgroups of patients, but even in these very large trials extreme caution is needed to interpret the results appropriately.

Subgroups and lunacy

Consider the classic example provided by the investigators of the ISIS-2 randomized trial of aspirin in acute MI. They demonstrated the unreliability of subgroup analyses by subdividing the clear overall result (804 vascular deaths in the aspirin group versus 1016 vascular deaths in the placebo group—$P < 0.000001$) by astrological 'birth signs'. Twelve absurd subgroups emerged. In some birth signs, the results for aspirin were about average and in some they were, just by chance, a bit better or a bit worse than average. Libra and Gemini were subgroups with the least promising results—for just these two birth signs, no fewer deaths occurred with aspirin than with placebo (Table 6).

It would obviously be unwise to conclude from this analysis that patients with acute MI born under Libra or Gemini are unlikely to benefit from aspirin. Yet subgroup analyses that are no more statistically reliable than these are frequently reported and accepted, with inappropriate effects on clinical practice. For example, the use of aspirin after transient ischaemic attacks was, until recently, approved in the USA for men but not for women because of selective emphasis on small subgroups in particular trials. In retrospect, this was a lethal mistake, resulting in many women being denied a life-saving treatment that produces about the same benefits for women as for men [1, 11].

Table 6 Example of a misleading subgroup analysis: false-negative mortality effect in a subgroup defined only by the astrological birth sign: the ISIS-2 (1988) trial of aspirin among over 17 000 acute MI patients [20].

Astrological birth sign	No. of 1-month deaths (aspirin vs placebo)	Statistical significance
Libra or Gemini	150 vs 147	NS
All other signs	654 vs 869	$2P < 0.000001$
Any birth sign[a]	804 vs 1016 (9.4%) (11.8%)	$2P < 0.000001$

[a]Appropriate overall analysis for assessing the true effect in all subgroups.

Interpretation of trials

The totality of evidence

Keep your feet on the ground

- Before changing your clinical behaviour in response to a particular trial, consider all other relevant randomized studies on that therapeutic question (or, even better, consult a well-conducted meta-analysis)
- Be wary of initial small trials with extreme findings; their apparent promise may be short-lived.

As described later, meta-analysis of all relevant trials on a therapeutic question is one way of reducing false-negative and false-positive results in particular studies. It is especially helpful when new trials report their findings in the context of an updated meta-analysis of previous trials.

For example, the placebo-controlled PEP study randomized 13 356 patients undergoing surgery for hip fracture to 160 mg aspirin daily, started preoperatively and continued for 35 days [12]. About 1.6% (105/6679) of the patients allocated aspirin had pulmonary embolism or deep venous thrombosis, compared with 2.5% (165/6677) allocated placebo. PEP's conclusions were reinforced by a meta-analysis of all previous relevant trials of aspirin, including data from about 9000 additional patients undergoing orthopaedic or general surgery or at high risk of venous thromboembolism for medical reasons.

What is a reasonable attitude to take when a small trial reports an extreme observation, but the total evidence on that therapeutic question is still sparse? In general, be sceptical. Small-scale randomized studies may provide misleading results not just of the size but also of the direction of the effects of treatment on major outcomes.

For example, it was concluded, from a randomized placebo-controlled trial among 500 patients with heart failure, that 60 mg daily of the inotropic agent vesnarinone more than halved the risk of death (33 placebo vs 13 vesnarinone deaths) [13]. By contrast, when the same regimen was studied in a much larger number of the same type of patients, mortality was significantly increased (242 placebo vs 292 vesnarinone deaths) [14].

There are many other examples of extreme observations from initial small trials not being confirmed by much larger randomized studies (see Further reading for additional examples).

Extrapolation

Is it relevant to my patient?

- It is usually necessary to apply information from trials to patients outside the trials, possibly with different characteristics from the study participants
- Appropriate extrapolation varies from situation to situation.

Participants in trials may be a skewed subset of the entire target population, e.g. participants are, by definition, volunteers who may be more health conscious than non-volunteers. Also, some trials involve only specific groups, such as men, white people, middle-aged people or those with previous disease. How can the findings of such studies be applied to groups outside the trials?

In these situations, it is important to note the distinction between:
- proportional benefits (such as a 40% proportional risk reduction, from 10% to 6%)
- absolute benefits (in the above example, 4% or 40 events avoided per 1000 treated).

When the proportional effect of treatment on some particular outcome appears to be about constant in different patients in trials, a reasonable policy of extrapolation is to apply the proportional reduction observed in the trials to the absolute risk of the outcome in the particular group outside the trial.

For example, a reduction in diastolic blood pressure of 5–6 mmHg achieved in trials of antihypertensive therapy produced proportional risk reductions of about 40% for stroke and 15% for coronary heart disease. Each of these proportional effects appeared to be similar among a broad range of individuals in Europe and North America [15]. How would these results be applied to people in Russia? The absolute risk of stroke and coronary heart disease is several times higher in Russia than in Western European countries. This implies that the absolute benefit of blood pressure lowering for vascular disease should be even greater among Russians than among Westerners, assuming that the proportional effects are similar in Russia to those in Western populations.

Meta-analysis of trials

Strengths and limitations

- A meta-analysis can provide a less biased, more precise and more detailed assessment of the available information on a topic than individual studies can
- The preferential publication of striking results in small studies ('publication bias') may skew meta-analyses
- The reliability of a meta-analysis depends on the quality and quantity of the data that go into it.

'Meta-analysis' refers to the practice of combining data. Its aim is to provide a more comprehensive assessment of a topic than individual studies can. However, not all meta-analyses of randomized trials are trustworthy. There are two main concerns:
- How carefully was the overview performed?
- How large is it?

The simplest approach is merely to collect and tabulate the published data from whatever randomized trial reports are easily accessible in the literature. This approach will, however, miss relevant trials, and the studies included may be unrepresentative as a result of the preferential publication of extremely promising or extremely pessimistic results ('publication bias').

At the opposite extreme, meta-analyses can make extensive efforts to locate every potentially relevant randomized trial in systematic searches of the published and unpublished medical literature (see Section 4), to seek individual data on each patient ever randomized into those trials, to check and correct the original data, and then to produce analyses in collaboration with the original trialists. When really large, such meta-analyses may actually provide statistically reliable subgroup analyses of the effect of treatment in particular types of patient.

The power of a well-conducted meta-analysis

Consider the Early Breast Cancer Trialists' Collaborative Group [16] ('early' breast cancer referring to disease limited to the breast and the locoregional lymph nodes, which can be removed surgically). Taken separately, most of the trials of adjuvant tamoxifen were too small to provide reliable evidence about long-term survival. However, when the original data of 55 trials involving about 37 000 women were combined in 1995, some very definite differences in 10-year survival emerged. For example, among women with potentially hormone-sensitive breast cancer, about 5 years of adjuvant tamoxifen treatment improved the 10-year survival rate from 66% to 74% (Fig. 8).

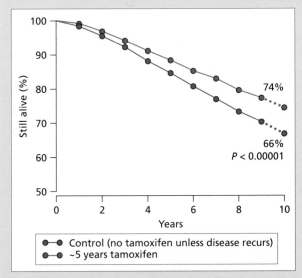

Fig. 8 Effects of hormonal adjuvant tamoxifen for early breast cancer on 10-year survival in a worldwide overview of randomized trials [16]. The graph shows the survival of all women with potentially hormone-sensitive breast cancer with and without tamoxifen.

Another important aspect of this meta-analysis was that it was large enough to look reliably at tamoxifen's effects in particular subgroups of women. Before this report, tamoxifen was not usually given to younger patients with early breast cancer because most clinicians did not believe that it helped premenopausal women. But the meta-analysis found that the proportional benefits of tamoxifen were similar in women irrespective of age, menopausal status, spread to the local lymph nodes or use of chemotherapy. The report concluded that another 20 000 lives each year could be saved worldwide if tamoxifen was given immediately after surgery to all breast cancer patients who needed it, regardless of age and other characteristics.

Interpreting 'forest plots'

 Meta-analyses often use diagrams, such as 'forest plots', to summarize large amounts of information.

Meta-analyses should aim to present information concisely and in an accessible way. The use of certain diagrams (sometimes called 'forest plots') can achieve both aims. There can be minor variations in the form of such plots in the medical literature, but the diagrams typically summarize key information in only a single row of a table from each of the studies in an overview. Plotting the results of individual studies on a common axis provides a convenient visual comparison of the separate trial results,

and a synthesis of the data can be shown graphically on the same plot.

As an example, consider the Antiplatelet Trialists' Collaboration [1], briefly mentioned at the start of this section. By 1994, this meta-analysis involved information from 145 randomized trials of aspirin or other antiplatelet therapies, mainly related to the secondary prevention of vascular disease. Fig. 9 shows just the 11 trials of antiplatelet regimens in patients with prior MI.

• A single row in the table summarizes information from a particular trial, including the drug regimen, numbers allocated to each treatment and the corresponding numbers of vascular events in each group.

• The horizontal axis of the graph represents the odds of avoiding death or recurrences of MI or stroke on antiplatelet treatment compared with control (an odds ratio of 1.0 indicates no difference whatsoever).

• Black squares represent odds ratios in each study, with the area of the square proportional to the number of events in each study, e.g. the AMIS study involves a larger number of vascular events than any of the other trials in the figure, so the area of its square is the largest.

• Horizontal lines emerging from the squares represent confidence intervals. Larger studies have narrower confidence intervals than smaller studies (and, once again, as a result of its size the AMIS study has the narrowest confidence interval of the 11 trials).

• In this example, the overall result and its confidence interval are indicated by an unshaded diamond. Note the

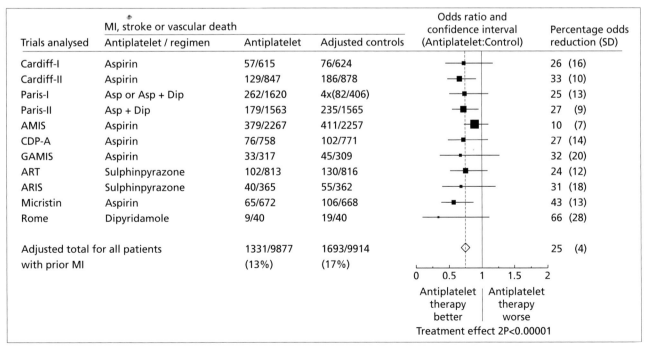

Trials analysed	MI, stroke or vascular death			Odds ratio and confidence interval (Antiplatelet:Control)	Percentage odds reduction (SD)
	Antiplatelet / regimen	Antiplatelet	Adjusted controls		
Cardiff-I	Aspirin	57/615	76/624		26 (16)
Cardiff-II	Aspirin	129/847	186/878		33 (10)
Paris-I	Asp or Asp + Dip	262/1620	4x(82/406)		25 (13)
Paris-II	Asp + Dip	179/1563	235/1565		27 (9)
AMIS	Aspirin	379/2267	411/2257		10 (7)
CDP-A	Aspirin	76/758	102/771		27 (14)
GAMIS	Aspirin	33/317	45/309		32 (20)
ART	Sulphinpyrazone	102/813	130/816		24 (12)
ARIS	Sulphinpyrazone	40/365	55/362		31 (18)
Micristin	Aspirin	65/672	106/668		43 (13)
Rome	Dipyridamole	9/40	19/40		66 (28)
Adjusted total for all patients with prior MI		1331/9877 (13%)	1693/9914 (17%)		25 (4)

Antiplatelet therapy better | Antiplatelet therapy worse
Treatment effect 2P<0.00001

Fig. 9 Meta-analysis of 11 randomized trials of prolonged antiplatelet therapy versus control in patients with prior myocardial infarction [1]. Test for heterogeneity: $\chi^2_{10} = 12.3$; $P > 0.1$; NS. Asp, aspirin; Dip, dipyridamole; MI, myocardial infarction.

diamond's narrow width. This indicates a high degree of precision as a result of the combination of the 11 separate results.

• Overall, the studies indicate a 25% reduction in vascular events among patients allocated antiplatelet treatment compared with those allocated control. The 'test for heterogeneity' indicates that there was no significant statistical scatter among the 11 separate results ($P > 0.1$).

This particular example demonstrates several of the advantages of meta-analysis. Taken separately, 8 of the 11 trials in Table 7 were too small to have yielded statistically reliable evidence on their own (as each of their confidence intervals was consistent with an odds ratio of 1.0).

Furthermore, in retrospect, the three other trials were significant only because, by chance, they had results that were too good to be true. By contrast, the overall result indicating a 25% reduction in vascular recurrences and death was clear and convincing ($P < 0.00001$).

Ethics in randomized trials

There must be sufficient doubt about a therapy to withhold it from half the patients in a trial, and at the same time there must be sufficient belief in the therapy's potential to justify giving it to the remaining half.

The Declaration of Helsinki has been accepted internationally as the basis for ethical clinical research. The rights of patients include: the liberty to abstain from a study; the provision of adequate information about potential benefits and potential hazards of involvement; the desirability of giving written consent before participation; and the freedom to withdraw from a study at any time. In the UK, investigators can submit research protocols for review to local research ethics committees or, in the case of multicentre trials, to a regional committee.

When randomized trials recruit patients according to the 'uncertainty principle', there is usually a reasonable parallel between good science and good ethics. This principle states that the fundamental criterion for eligibility is that both patient and doctor should be substantially uncertain about the appropriateness of each of the trial treatments for that particular patient [17]. If there are strong preferences for one or another treatment (by either the patient or the doctor), then that patient is ineligible. However, if both parties are substantially uncertain, randomization is appropriate.

Do you need an operation on your carotids?

The European Carotid Surgery Trial compared a policy of immediate carotid endarterectomy with a policy of 'watchful waiting' in 3000 patients with partial carotid artery stenosis and a recent transient ischaemic attack [18]. There were substantial differences between clinicians in the types of patients they were prepared to randomize, particularly in terms of severity of carotid stenosis. As recruitment in the trial was based on the uncertainty principle, this diversity of opinions ensured representation from each patient category, including mild, moderate and severe stenosis. The study was therefore able to provide direct evidence in each case, demonstrating clear benefits of immediate surgery for patients with severe stenosis (70–99%), uncertain benefits for patients with moderate stenosis (30–69%) and net hazards for patients with mild stenosis (0–29%).

Abbreviated references

1 *BMJ* 1994; 308: 81.
2 *Lancet* 1995; 345: 669.
3 *Lancet* 1988; ii: 349.
4 *N Engl J Med* 2000; 342: 145.
5 *Lancet* 1994; 344: 1383.
6 *JAMA* 1982; 248: 1465.
7 *Paediatrics* 1989; 84: 957.
8 *Lancet* 1996; 348: 75.
9 *N Engl J Med* 1980; 303: 1038.
10 *Lancet* 2000; 355: 766.
11 *Federal Register* 1998; 63: 56802.
12 *Lancet* 2000; 355: 1295.
13 *N Engl J Med* 1993; 329: 149.
14 *N Engl J Med* 1998; 339: 1810.
15 *Lancet* 1990; 335: 827.
16 *Lancet* 1998; 351: 1451.
17 Weatherall DJ, Ledingham JGG, Warrell DA, eds. *Oxford Textbook of Medicine*, 3rd edn. Oxford: Oxford University Press, 1996: 21.
18 *Lancet* 1991; 337: 1235.

Further reading

Collins R, MacMahon S. Reliable assessment of the effects of treatment on mortality and major morbidity. *Lancet* 2001; 357: 373–380.
Collins R, Peto R, Gray R, Parish S. Large-scale randomized evidence: trials and overviews. In: Weatherall DJ, Ledingham JGG, Warrell DA, eds. *Oxford Textbook of Medicine*, 3rd edn. Oxford: Oxford University Press, 1996: 21–32.
Peto R *et al.* Design and analysis of randomized clinical trials requiring prolonged observation of each patient (Parts I and II). *Br J Cancer* 1976; 34: 585–612; 1977; 35: 1–39.
Hennekens CH, Buring JE. *Epidemiology in Medicine.* Boston: Little & Brown, 1987.
Pocock SJ. *Clinical Trials: A Practical Approach.* New York: John Wiley & Sons, 1983.

4 Evidence-based medicine

Defining evidence-based medicine

> Evidence-based medicine is the explicit and judicious integration of clinical expertise, valid external evidence and patient preferences in determining medical practice [1] (Fig. 10).

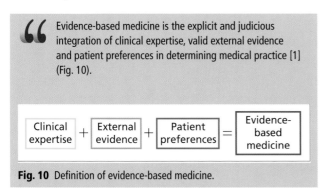

Fig. 10 Definition of evidence-based medicine.

- By clinical expertise, we mean the ability to use clinical skills and past experience to formulate diagnoses and provide treatment rapidly. This also involves the ability to communicate, e.g. present the individual risks and benefits of potential interventions to patients, acknowledging their personal values and expectations.
- By valid external evidence, we mean clinically relevant research, especially that into the accuracy and precision of diagnostic tests (including the clinical examination), the power of prognostic markers, and the efficacy and safety of therapeutic, rehabilitative and preventive regimens. New evidence from clinical research can both invalidate previously accepted diagnostic tests and treatments and replace them with new ones that are more powerful, more accurate, more efficacious and safer.
- By patient preferences we mean the unique values, concerns and expectations that each patient brings to a clinical encounter, which must be integrated into clinical decisions if they are to serve the patient.

Evidence-based medicine (EBM) neither undervalues clinical expertise and experience nor overvalues the findings of valid research. By integrating patient preferences, it aims to be founded on evidence and responsive to individual patients' choices.

How evidence-based medicine differs from traditional approaches

The concepts of EBM are not new. The application of the principles of science to medicine found expression in post-revolutionary Paris, when clinicians such as Pierre Louis rejected the pronouncements of authorities (such as Louis's rejection of the dictate that venesection was good for cholera!) and sought the truth through systematic observation

of patients. These principles may be traced further back to ancient Chinese medicine where, during the reign of Emperor Qianlong, the method of '*kaozheng*' ('practising evidential research') was used to interpret ancient Confucian texts (J. Woodhouse, personal communication, 1998). In the current era they were consolidated and in 1992 they were named EBM by a group led by Gordon Guyatt at McMaster University in Canada [2].

Detractors have argued that there is nothing new about EBM [3], but it has gained many advocates, and many clinicians have made good use of some of the advantages offered by EBM [4]. Whether it differs from more traditional approaches hardly matters: EBM is vindicated by its ability to offer an explicit and accessible route to the practice of clinical medicine, based on the findings of valid research and cognisant of patients' wishes. The differences between EBM and more traditional approaches are summarized in Table 7.

Table 7 Differences between evidence-based medicine (EBM) and traditional approaches.

EBM	Traditional approaches
Explicit and accessible	Can be élitist and obscure
Makes use of rigid tuition aids to identify clinical questions within clinical cases	Emphasizes free-form 'think for yourself'
Structures clinical questions to identify appropriate: research methodologies sources of evidence searching terms	No clear link between bedside and library
Makes optimal use of: library skills and evidence retrieval modern electronic libraries	Accessing evidence is not formally taught Sources of evidence rarely explained
Employs explicit guides to critical appraisal	No formal guidelines for critical appraisal
Requires practitioners to integrate external evidence with patient choices	Patient choice sometimes considered

Evidence-based medicine specifically acknowledges four problems and has been made possible by recent developments. The following are the realizations:
- The need for valid information about diagnosis, prognosis, therapy and prevention (up to five times per inpatient [5] and twice for every three outpatients [6]).

• The inadequacy of traditional sources for this information because they are out of date (textbooks [7]), frequently wrong (experts [8]), ineffective (didactic continuing medical education [9]), or too overwhelming in their volume and too variable in their validity for practical clinical use (medical journals [10]).

• The disparity between our diagnostic skills and clinical judgement, which increase with experience, and our up-to-date knowledge [11] and clinical performance [12], which tend to decline.

• Our inability to afford more than a few seconds per patient for finding and assimilating this evidence [13], or to set aside more than half an hour per week for general reading and study [14].

Until recently, these problems were insurmountable in full-time clinical practice. However, five developments have changed this situation:

1 The development of strategies for efficiently retrieving and appraising evidence (for its validity, impact and relevance) [15].

2 The creation of systematic reviews and concise summaries of the effects of health care (epitomized by the Cochrane Collaboration [16]).

3 The creation of evidence-based journals of secondary publication (which publish the 2% of clinical articles that are both valid and of immediate clinical use [17]).

4 The creation of information systems for bringing the foregoing to us in seconds [10].

5 The identification and application of effective strategies for life-long learning and for improving our clinical performance [18].

What is new about EBM?

• Strategies for finding and using evidence
• Systematic reviews
• Journals of secondary publication
• Informatics resources and software that allow the rapid and accurate handling of evidence
• The use of EBM to integrate continuing professional development into service delivery.

EBM in practice

Evidence-based medicine can be used in daily practice as a framework for clinical management.
(Rosenberg [19])

Away from the bedside, systematic analyses can be performed using EBM to determine best practice and to draw up guidelines and protocols. Clinical governance requires individual practitioners to be capable of distinguishing good practice from bad. This process is aided by the use of structured, explicit and agreed methodologies for distinguishing best from inadequate practice.

In the field of health policy, EBM has triggered the development of evidence-based health care [20] and the precepts of EBM are being used by the National Institute for Clinical Excellence (NICE) and other bodies established to ensure that clinical practice reflects knowledge of the most effective interventions.

Finally, and the purpose of this section of the *Medical Masterclass*, EBM is being used as a framework for problem-based education [21], teaching generic skills that encourage life-long learning.

Four steps in the practice of evidence-based medicine

Four key steps to EBM

1 Question formulation
2 Finding evidence
3 Critical appraisal
4 Application of the evidence to clinical care

The practice of EBM involves four integrated steps:

• Step 1: converting the need for information (about prevention, diagnosis, prognosis, therapy, causation, etc.) into an answerable question.

• Step 2: finding the best evidence with which to answer that question.

• Step 3: critically appraising that evidence for its validity (proximity to the truth), impact (size of the effect) and applicability (usefulness in the care of specific patients).

• Step 4: integrating the findings of the critical appraisal with clinical findings and the individual circumstances of the patient.

Step 1: Question formulation

This involves converting the need for information (about prevention, diagnosis, prognosis, therapy, causation, etc.) into an answerable question. Clinical cases often encompass many different clinical problems, each of which might generate several questions. Without a structure we might be tempted to ask questions to which we already know the answers, or alternatively questions that interest us the most, rather than those most likely to benefit the patient. EBM provides a structure that can be used to identify the key components of a clinical problem, which can then be used to ask a question that has a high probability of securing an answer, i.e. an answerable question.

Key elements of an answerable question

To be answerable a question must be focused and should include each of the following four elements:

1 A patient or problem: defined by specific characteristics that are likely to influence the applicability of the evidence. Thus, an exercise tolerance ECG, although informative about angina in a middle-aged man, is likely to be considerably less accurate in helping you to diagnose cardiac ischaemia in an elderly woman.

2 An intervention: this might be a diagnostic test, a therapeutic intervention or information concerning prognosis.

3 A comparison: in questions about diagnosis this might be a well-established test; for treatment, it might be placebo or an alternative treatment.

4 Outcome measures: it is vital to identify outcome measures that are clinically important to you and your patient, rather than those that are easily measured. Thus angina, re-infarction and death are more important than thallium scan measurements; bone pain and fracture rates are more important than changes in DEXA scan readings.

Questions can arise in a large number of domains:
- Diagnosis
- Treatment
- Prognosis
- Aetiology
- Health economics
- Harm
- Clinical skills
- Education.

The nature of the question, both the element and domain, will determine the most appropriate research methodology to be employed in generating valid evidence. Although randomized controlled trials provide the most reliable evidence about therapies, prospective cohort studies with good follow-up will provide valid evidence about prognosis.

 The Cochrane Database of Systematic Reviews contains high-quality evidence about treatment. It will not be a good source for evidence about prognosis, which might be more readily accessed through a search of the primary literature on MEDLINE.

Advantages of posing answerable questions

Why bother formulating questions clearly? There are no controlled trials that demonstrate that doing so leads to better evidence, found faster, and used more wisely in patient care—although this was suggested by a randomized controlled trial of teaching question formulation with searching skills [22].

Those who use question formulation as part of their clinical practice cite seven advantages to focused questions:

1 They help make the optimal use of scarce time by focusing on evidence that is directly relevant to the patients' clinical needs.

2 They help make optimal use of our scarce educational time by helping us select evidence that directly addresses our particular knowledge needs, or those of our learners.

3 They can be used to identify terms that will enhance our ability to search for evidence most effectively (see below).

4 They help us identify the domain of the question, and thus the most appropriate research methodology used to generate the evidence that will help us answer the question.

5 They help us communicate effectively with our colleagues by requiring us to identify the specific issues relating to individual patients.

6 They can provide a framework for teaching and learning which can be easily shared, modelled and used for life-long learning.

7 Answering questions is always satisfying, often generates further questions and helps us resolve problems more rapidly.

 The benefits of a well-formed question
- Focus on relevant problems
- Help us make optimal use of time
- Can be used to identify search terms
- Suggest appropriate research methodology by identifying the domain of the question
- Help us communicate with our colleagues
- Creates a framework for teaching
- Helps identify areas of uncertainty and learning needs.

Problems in posing answerable questions

Question formulation is the single aspect of EBM with which practitioners find the greatest difficulty. Three problems often impede the posing of answerable questions:

1 Identifying questions to which we do not know the answers.

2 Articulating the questions.

3 Having more than one question to answer.

There can be uncertainty over whether a clinical problem contains questions to which we do not know the answers (as we all prefer to hide our ignorance!). Asking ourselves whether we can cover all domains relating to any particular clinical problem will help identify unseen questions. Do we know what the prognosis is in this condition? How does one treatment compare with another? Too often we regard the identification of a gap in our knowledge as ignorance rather than a learning opportunity. The former response works to the detriment of ourselves and our patients, whereas the latter may benefit both.

All of us will sometimes have difficulty in articulating a question. When this happens, using the rigid structure of the four elements of an answerable question will often help to focus on the issue (or in most people's experience the issues) at hand.

The four elements of an answerable question

Which of the following do we need to address:
1 A patient or problem
2 An intervention
3 A comparison
4 Outcome measures.

Often we have more questions than time. This will almost always be the case, so we need to develop a strategy for deciding where to begin. Learning occurs in many small increments over a long time and attempts to do it all at once are impossible and therefore bound to frustrate.

Problems that impede the posing of answerable questions include:
• uncertainty over our own knowledge and ignorance
• difficulty in identifying and articulating a question
• more questions than time
• fear of questions.

Factors to consider when deciding which question to answer first include:
• Which question is most important to the patient's well-being?
• Which question is most likely to recur in our practice?
• Which question is most relevant to our learners' needs?
• Which question is most feasible to answer within the time we have available?
• Which question is most interesting?

Step 2: Finding evidence

The second step is to find the best evidence with which to answer the question that has been posed. Searching for evidence is not an intuitive skill: a randomized controlled trial has shown that students taught how to search are more effective searchers than their untutored peers [22].

The following are the key elements of effective searching:
• Knowledge of the question
• Knowledge of the existing available sources of evidence
• Recognition of which sources are likely to contain the evidence most likely to answer the question
• Knowledge of how to search for the evidence in the relevant sources, including the structure of databases, relevant search terms and methodological filters.

It is beyond the scope of this text to describe searching strategies in detail [1]. Two types of sources deserve specific mention because of their usefulness and the frequency with which they are used by physicians:
• MEDLINE
• EBM journals.

MEDLINE

MEDLINE is the database compiled by librarians in the National Library of Medicine in Bethesda, Maryland, USA. It is divided into sections labelled with 'medical subheadings' (MeSH), into which all indexed publications are placed. Within each MeSH category, indexed publications are tagged with tabs or labels designating terms that describe the nature of the publication and specific words contained within the text. In addition, a label describing the nature of the published material (such as 'Randomized controlled trial' or 'Meta-analysis') is added.

Searching software packages such as SilverPlatter's WinSpirs enable searchers to select articles in specific categories, bearing selected tabs or labels. Search terms can be combined or excluded using 'Boolian' terms (AND, OR, NOT) and a search can be restricted using terms that 'limit' the search by year of publication, language, publication type and a number of other terms. Without training it is impossible to take full advantage of the power of searching software or to make optimal use of electronic databases such as MEDLINE.

EBM journals

MEDLINE and WinSpirs represent technically exacting and precise ways for searching the primary literature. This method of accessing sources of evidence is time-consuming but, when used correctly, is likely to yield the best available evidence. However, those working in 'front-line' clinical jobs often do not have the time to conduct searches of this type; an alternative approach is provided by evidence-based journals and online service.

Beginning with the *American College of Physicians (ACP) Journal Club* in 1991, a growing number of periodicals summarize the best evidence in traditional journals, making their selections according to explicit criteria for validity, impact and interest, providing structured abstracts of the best studies, and expert commentaries to provide the context of the studies and the clinical applicability of their findings. These new journals include:
• *Evidence-Based Medicine*
• *Evidence-Based Health Care Policy and Practice*
• *Evidence-Based Cardiovascular Medicine*.

These journals select the very best articles published in a wide range of primary journals and so provide rapid access to the best evidence. When these sources yield evidence they are reliable, but they are not a panacea:

• because most of these journals are in their infancy, they contain a restricted volume of evidence

• because, although they cover mainstream topics in depth, coverage is less complete or non-existent in specialist areas.

These deficits can be overcome by requesting the title pages of key journals from services such as Current Contents, MEDLINE and SilverPlatter—but here again we run into the problem of time.

 ScHARR provides excellent links to evidence-based services: www.shef.ac.uk/uni/academic/R-Z/scharr/ir/netting.html

Step 3: Critical appraisal

 Key questions addressed in critical appraisal
- Is the study valid?
- Are the results important?
- Is the evidence applicable to my patients?

As with searching, critical appraisal skills are not acquired without study and practice, but critical appraisal is so essential to the process of making the best use of evidence that time spent mastering these skills is well rewarded. Critical appraisal teaching has been developed and refined for groups ranging from trained clinical epidemiologists to the lay public. The Evidence Based Medicine Working Party in McMaster developed 'Users' Guides to the Medical Literature' which were published in the *Journal of the American Medical Association* in 1992. These guides have been reproduced in numerous later publications but have not been improved upon. Having identified relevant evidence it must be appraised for its:

• validity (closeness to the truth)

• importance (size of the effect)

• applicability (usefulness in our clinical practice).

Validity

Specific guides can be used rapidly to determine the validity of an article; these address such issues as:

• Are the aims of the study clearly stated?

• Is the methodology appropriate for the aim of the study?

• Are the data analysed appropriately?

Articles failing criteria for validity can be rejected and the search can continue. Valid articles can be appraised for the importance of the results.

Importance

There are no objective guides that will help us decide what is and what is not important. In each case we make

our own judgement, but biostatistical methods can be used (e.g. absolute risk reduction, the risk ratio, odds ratios and the number needed to treat—see Section 1, p. 6) to provide a common determinant that can be used to compare different studies. Some understanding of the statistical tests used to determine significance and precision is useful when reading the results sections of articles. However, too often we trust the editorial staff of the journals to reject reports of findings that are not significant or results that are wildly imprecise (wide confidence intervals).

Applicability

The third element of critical appraisal requires that we consider whether valid and important results are applicable to particular patients. Crucial differences between the subjects included in clinical trials and the patients whom we encounter may tempt us to discount articles that we would otherwise value. Before rejecting important findings of valid studies, it is worth performing what is known in the jargon as a sensitivity analysis:

• Consider how much difference it might make if our patient was only half as likely as the trial subjects to respond to a treatment. If such a patient would derive a significant benefit from the treatment, then the study is still valid.

• Consider also how much difference it might make if our patient was perhaps twice as likely as the trial subjects to suffer a side effect of treatment. Would the 85-year-old man with atrial fibrillation who keeps falling over really be well served by anticoagulation?

Step 4: Application of the evidence to clinical care

Application to clinical care involves integrating the critical appraisal of the evidence with our clinical expertise and with our patient's specific circumstances. Evidence, no matter how valid and important, is referable to the subjects of the studies that generate that evidence. To determine the applicability of evidence to the needs of our patients, the use of clinical expertise is required to:

• elucidate clinical symptoms and signs

• identify the patient's specific ideas, concerns and expectations

• determine how these attributes differ from those of the patients in the clinical studies.

Even when evidence is widely known and well understood it cannot be used indiscriminately. Consider the use of β blockers for mild heart failure. Although evidence of their beneficial effect is now well established, the clinician must be able to distinguish moderate from severe heart failure, identify symptoms and signs that might contraindicate their use, and communicate the risks and benefits of their use to the patient. At this stage patient preferences can be used to weight evidence. Although β blockers may be indicated as an effective treatment for mild heart failure, having heard of the side effects a patient may refuse this therapy in favour of a diuretic, preferring the less effective but still beneficial therapy because of its better profile of adverse actions. Medicine is about helping patients to make such informed choices.

Can evidence-based medicine be used by clinicians?

In a survey of UK GPs (in which over half the responders held the MRCP), the great majority reported that they practised 'searching', using evidence-based summaries generated by others (72%) and evidence-based practice guidelines or protocols (84%) [23]. However, far fewer claimed to understand (and be able to explain) the 'appraising' tools of NNTs (35%) and confidence intervals (20%).

Despite the fact that the majority used some of the key steps of EBM, only 5% believed that learning the skills of evidence-based medicine, i.e. to identify and appraise the primary literature or systematic reviews oneself, was the most appropriate method for 'moving from opinion-based medicine to evidence-based general practice'. This may at least in part indicate a difference of opinion over terminology, something that is rife regarding EBM.

Rapidly accessing EBM

Can evidence be accessed rapidly enough to have an impact in clinical practice? It appears so. When a busy (180+ admissions per month) inpatient medical service brought electronic summaries of evidence previously appraised either by team members (critically appraised topics or CATs) or by the summary journals to working rounds, it was documented that, on average, the former could be accessed in 10 s and the latter in 25 s [10]. Moreover, when assessed from the viewpoint of the most junior member of the team caring for the patient, this evidence changed 25% of their diagnostic and treatment suggestions and added to a further 23% of them.

Evidence appraisal

• CATs, or critically appraised topics, are one-page summaries of the practice of question formulation, searching and critical appraisal

• *Best Evidence* is an electronic version of the two journals of secondary publication, *ACP Journal Club* and *Evidence Based Medicine*.

Translating evidence into clinical practice

When they can find evidence, can clinicians actually provide evidence-based care to their patients? Again, it appears so from audits carried out on clinical services that attempt to operate in the searching and appraising modes. The first of these examined the evidence base for the primary interventions applied to the primary diagnoses of consecutive patients on an inpatient medical service. This documented that 82% of primary interventions were evidence based: 53% were based on randomized trials or systematic reviews of randomized trials and 29% on convincing non-experimental evidence [24]. Similar results have been obtained from audits of psychiatric [25], surgical [26], paediatric [27] and general [28] practice. In each case, the denominator used was the number of patients admitted, not the number of different diagnoses; evidence is available for far fewer diagnoses than clinical cases.

Our daily clinical experience might lead us to ask questions about treatment for one patient with a rare vasculitic eye problem for which no therapeutic trials exist, five patients with myocardial ischaemia and two with cerebrovascular accidents. Good quality evidence can be found for seven of the eight patients but for only two thirds of the diagnoses.

Practising evidence-based medicine

Evidence-based medicine is practised in many different environments. Some examples of successful practice by clinicians are described below.

On the ward or in the clinic

When clinical problems are encountered as part of daily clinical work, questions will arise that can be either ignored or addressed. One technique for capturing questions is to use 'educational prescriptions', in which a clinical scenario is described and a question identified.

The educational prescription

1 Time, date and place
2 Name of learner
3 Four-part question: a patient or problem; an intervention; a comparison; outcome measures
4 Time, place and date at which script is to be filled
5 Name of teacher issuing script.

A member of the clinical team, often ourselves, is issued with the educational prescription that describes the question identifying a learning need. The prescription also states the time and place at which it should be 'filled' and thus it represents a learning contract.

Some baulk at the style and formality of this device, but essentially it says: 'this is the question—when can we talk about the answer(s), if there are any?' During schooldays, the term 'homework' described something similar and, as with homework, less experienced learners may benefit from some guidance in how and where to search for evidence and the critical appraisal of the evidence.

The team/firm meeting

Physicians can adapt clinical team meetings to incorporate EBM. One method is as follows: in the first part of a meeting a clinical case is presented, following which a clinical question is formulated. A member of the team is delegated, retrieving an article that is then critically appraised at the next team meeting. After the critical appraisal, the team decides how to use the evidence in their future clinical practice. In the jargon, this completes the EBM group learning cycle.

The EBM group learning cycle

1 Clinical case presentation
2 Question formulation
3 (Search takes place away from the meeting)
4 Critical appraisal of relevant papers (including feedback on how search was performed)
5 Debate about application of evidence to the group's clinical practice
6 Possible creation of a guideline or protocol, or plan for research if evidence is lacking.

The journal club

It has been argued that we are irresponsible if we allow the postman to dictate the agenda for a journal club. Selecting the most relevant papers from the journals that come through our letterboxes does not ensure that our most pressing educational needs are met.

The format of a journal club can be changed by identifying dominant learning needs, ranking them in order, and then formulating specific questions to be answered. Members of the journal club select the questions that they wish to answer and then search for the best available journal articles. This search is not restricted to recent publications or even specific journals. The only determinants governing the search for evidence are that the evidence should be relevant and valid. These articles then form the subject of the journal club, ensuring that the articles discussed are directly relevant to the team's clinical practice. Critical appraisal during the journal club follows the steps and questions in the users' guides to the medical literature.

Does providing evidence-based care improve outcomes for patients?

No such evidence is available from randomized trials because no investigative team or research-granting agency has yet overcome the problems of sample size, contamination, blinding and long-term follow-up that such a trial requires. Moreover, there are ethical concerns with such a trial: is withholding access to evidence from the control clinicians ethical? On the other hand, population-based 'outcomes research' has repeatedly documented that those patients who do receive evidence-based therapies have better outcomes than those who do not.

For positive examples, myocardial infarction survivors prescribed aspirin or β blockers have lower mortality rates than those who are not prescribed these drugs [29, 30] and, where clinicians use more warfarin and stroke unit referrals, the stroke mortality rate declines by >20% [31].

For a negative example, patients undergoing carotid surgery despite failing to meet evidence-based operative criteria, when compared with operated patients who meet those criteria, are more than three times as likely to suffer major stroke or death in the next month [32].

Whether these examples can be considered to represent the practice of EBM or merely good practice might be debated. Here we run into semantic issues again, but it is fair to argue that the wider dissemination of the results of trials, awareness of their existence and comprehension of their findings are all consequences of the practice of what is commonly known as EBM.

Limitations of evidence-based medicine

The examination of the concepts and practice of EBM has led to negative as well as positive reactions. The ensuing debate has identified three limitations that are universal to science and medicine:
• Shortage of clear and consistent scientific evidence
• Difficulties in applying any evidence to the care of individual patients
• Barriers to the practice of high-quality medicine.

The debate has also identified three limitations that are unique to the practice of EBM [33,34]:

1 The need to acquire new skills in question formulation, searching and critical appraisal can be daunting and is undoubtedly time-consuming. However, once learned, these skills are readily retained and if only the first two steps have been mastered evidence-based care can still be applied if the question and search are directed towards pre-appraised resources.

2 Clinicians have limited time to master and apply these new skills, and the resources required for instant access to evidence are often inadequate in clinical settings. However, with each passing week computers become more

widely dispersed and access to databases and electronic format journals becomes easier.

3 Evidence that EBM 'works' has been late and slow to come in some settings and is not available in others.

Limitations of EBM

1 Universal to science and medicine:
• shortage of clear, concise evidence
• difficulties in applying evidence
• barriers to practice.
2 Specific to EBM:
• need to acquire the new skills of EBM
• lack of time
• lack of evidence of effectiveness of EBM.

Misunderstandings about evidence-based medicine

Much discussion and debate has proposed bogus limitations of EBM which arise from misunderstandings. These misunderstandings may have arisen as a result either of errors of presentation by some exponents of EBM or of failure of some 'opponents' to read what was actually written, leading them to focus specifically on particular aspects that they elevated out of all proportion and then sought to demolish. Most probably, misunderstanding arose for both of these reasons.

An examination of the definition and steps of EBM, as explained in this module of the *Medical Masterclass*, should quickly dismiss the criticisms that it denigrates clinical expertise, is limited to clinical research, ignores patients' values and preferences, or promotes a 'cookbook' approach to medicine.

Other misunderstandings include the following:
• EBM is something forced on doctors by those who would seek to restrain the costs of health care. It is not necessarily an effective cost-cutting tool, because providing evidence-based care directed at maximizing patients' quality of life often increases costs and raises the ire of health economists [35].
• EBM only works in ivory towers, but the self-reported employment of the 'searching' mode by a great majority of 'front-line' GPs dispels this contention.
• EBM leads to therapeutic nihilism whenever there is no randomized trial evidence—this is nonsense; pragmatism requires that we find solutions to our patients' problems even when the best-available evidence is suboptimal. Should there be no evidence from randomized controlled trials, it is much better to base decisions on evidence from clinical experience or a case series than on guesswork or prejudice.

Other uses of evidence-based medicine

The other uses of EBM include the following.
• It reinforces the need for, and mastery of, the clinical and communication skills that are required to gather and critically appraise patients' stories, symptoms and signs, and to identify and incorporate their values and expectations when planning clinical management.
• It fosters generic skills for use in finding, appraising and implementing evidence from the basic sciences and other applied sciences.
• It provides an effective, efficient framework for postgraduate education and self-directed, life-long learning; when coupled with 'virtual libraries' and distance learning programmes, it supplies a model of worldwide applicability.
• Although not its primary aim, by identifying the questions for which there is no satisfactory evidence it generates a supremely pragmatic agenda for applied health research (i.e. formally recognized by groups such as the UK NHS R&D programme).
• It provides a common language for use by the multidisciplinary teams whose effective collaboration is essential if patients are to benefit from new knowledge.

Other uses of EBM

• Reinforces the need for clinical and communication skills
• Develops generic educational skills
• Forms a framework for life-long learning
• Identifies areas where further research is needed
• Unites health-care workers from different professions and specialties by using a common approach and language.

1 Sackett DL, Strauss S, Richardson WS, Rosenberg WM, Haynes RB. *Evidence Based Medicine. How to Practise and Teach,* 2nd edn. London: Churchill Livingstone, 2000.
2 Evidence-Based Medicine Working Group. Evidence-based medicine. A new approach to teaching the practice of medicine. *JAMA* 1992; 268: 2420–5.
3 Grahame-Smith DG. Clinical academic medicine: a Socratic dialogue. *BMJ* 1997; 315: 593–5.
4 Sackett DL, Rosenberg WM, Gray JA, Haynes RB, Richardson WS. Evidence based medicine: what it is and what it isn't. *BMJ* 1996; 312: 71–2.
5 Osheroff JA, Forsythe DE, Buchanan BG, Bankowitz RA, Blumenfeld BH, Miller RA. Physicians' information needs: analysis of questions posed during clinical teaching. *Ann Intern Med* 1991; 114: 576–81.
6 Covell DG, Uman GC, Manning PR. Information needs in office practice: are they being met? *Ann Intern Med* 1985; 103: 596–9.
7 Antman EM, Lau J, Kupelnick B, Mosteller F, Chalmers TC. A comparison of results of meta-analyses of randomised control trials and recommendations of clinical experts. *JAMA* 1992; 268: 240–8.

8   Oxman A, Guyatt GH. The science of reviewing research. *Ann NY Acad Sci* 1993; 703: 125–34.

9   Davis DA, Thomson MA, Oxman AD, Haynes RB. Changing physician performance: a systematic review of the effect of continuing medical education strategies. *JAMA* 1997; 274: 700–5.

10 Haynes RB. Where's the meat in clinical journals? [Editorial] *ACP Journal Club* 1993; 119: A22–3.

11 Evans CE, Haynes RB, Birkett NJ *et al.* Does a mailed continuing education program improve clinician performance? Results of a randomised trial in antihypertensive care. *JAMA* 1986; 255: 501–4.

12 Sackett DL, Haynes RB, Taylor DW, Gibson ES, Roberts RS, Johnson AL. Clinical determinants of the decision to treat primary hypertension. *Clin Res* 1977; 24: 648.

13 Sackett DL, Straus SE. Finding and applying evidence during clinical rounds: the 'evidence cart'. *JAMA* 1998; 280: 1336–8.

14 Sackett DL. Using evidence-based medicine to help physicians keep up-to-date. *Serials* 1997; 9: 178–81.

15 Sackett DL, Richardson WS, Rosenberg W, Haynes RB. *Evidence-based Medicine. How to Practise and Teach EBM.* London: Churchill-Livingstone, 1997.

16 *The Cochrane Library, Issue 2*. Oxford: Update Software, 1999.

17 At the time of writing, this list comprised (in order of first publication) *ACP Journal Club, Evidence-Based Medicine, Evidence-Based Health Policy and Management, Evidence-Based Cardiovascular Medicine, Evidence-Based Mental Health, Evidence-Based Nursing,* and a growing number of 'best-evidence' departments in existing journals.

18 Cochrane Effective Practice and Organisation of Care Group. *The Cochrane Library, Issue 2*. Oxford: Update Software, 1999.

19 Rosenberg W, Donald A. evidence based medicine: an approach to clinical problem-solving. *BMJ* 1995; 310: 1122–6.

20 Muir Gray JA. *Evidence-based Healthcare*. London: Churchill Livingstone, 1997.

21 Strauss S, Sackett D, Richardson S, Rosenberg WM, Haynes B. *A Seven Step Course in Evidence Based Medicine.* Oxford: Radcliffe Press, 1998.

22 Rosenberg WMC, Deeks J, Lusher A, Snowball R, Dooley G, Sackett D. Improving searching skills and evidence retrieval. *J R Coll Physicians, London* 1998; 32: 557–63.

23 McColl A, Smith H, White P, Field J. General practitioners' perceptions of the route to evidence based medicine: a questionnaire survey. *BMJ* 1998; 316: 361–5.

24 Ellis J, Mulligan I, Rowe J, Sackett DL. Inpatient general medicine is evidence based. *Lancet* 1995; 346: 407–10.

25 Geddes JR, Game D, Jenkins NE, Peterson LA, Pottinger GR, Sackett DL. In-patient psychiatric care is evidence-based. In: *Proceedings of the Royal College Psychiatrists 'Winter Meeting Stratford, UK,* January 1996; 23: 5.

26 Howes N, Chagla L, Thorpe M, McCulloch P. Surgical practice is evidence based. *Br J Surg* 1997; 84: 1220–3.

27 Kenny SE, Shankar KR, Rintala R, Lamont GL, Lloyd DA. Evidence-based surgery: interventions in a regional paediatric surgical unit. *Arch Dis Child* 1997; 76: 50–3.

28 Gill P, Dowell AC, Neal RD, Smith N, Heywood P, Wilson AE. Evidence based general practice: a retrospective study of interventions in one training practice. *BMJ* 1996; 312: 819–21.

29 Krumholz HM, Radford MJ, Ellerbeck EF *et al.* Aspirin for secondary prevention after acute myocardial infarction in the elderly: prescribed use and outcomes. *Ann Intern Med* 1996; 124: 292–8.

30 Krumholz HM, Radford MJ, Wang Y, Chen J, Heiat A, Marciniak TA. National use and effectiveness of beta-blockers for the treatment of elderly patients after acute myocardial infarction. National Cooperative Cardiovascular Project. *JAMA* 1998; 280: 623–9.

31 Mitchell JB, Ballard DJ, Whisnant JP, Ammering CJ, Samsa GP, Matchar DB. What role do neurologists play in determining the costs and outcomes of stroke patients? *Stroke* 1996; 27: 1937–43.

32 Wong JH, Findlay JM, Suarez-Almazor ME. Regional performance of carotid endarterectomy appropriateness, outcomes and risk factors for complications. *Stroke* 1997; 28: 891–8.

33 Sackett DL, Rosenberg WMC, Gray JAM, Haynes RB, Richardson WS. Evidence based medicine: what it is and what it isn't. *BMJ* 1996; 312: 71–2.

34 Straus SE, McAlister FA. The limitations of evidence-based medicine (in press).

35 Maynard A. Evidence-based medicine: an incomplete method for informing treatment choices. *Lancet* 1997; 349: 126–8.

5 Self-assessment

Answers are on pp. 95–97.

Question 1
In the field of statistics, which of the following statements regarding a forest plot is true?
A the area of the squares is proportional to the number of events in each study
B the lengths of the horizontal lines emerging from the squares represent standard deviations
C the lengths of the horizontal lines emerging from the squares represent two standard deviations
D the area of the squares is proportional to the magnitude of the treatment effect in each study
E it is a method of combining data when individual studies are of insufficient power to show an effect

Question 2
In the field of statistics, a factorial trial means that:
A two or more treatments are tested sequentially
B two or more treatments are tested simultaneously
C the patients in the trial are stratified into two or more groups
D each patient receives one active drug and one placebo treatment
E the trial takes more than one factor into account

Question 3
The following is a description of a test. "The new test has a sensitivity of 99% and a specificity of 83%. In those under 65 years old it has a positive predictive value of 48%". A test with these characteristics would NOT be appropriate in which one of the following situations?
A rapid screening for HIV in a same-day-result STI clinic
B screening anonymously donated blood for HIV before transfusion
C as a preliminary part of a medical assessment looking for heart disease in potential army recruits
D a screening test for head lice in children
E as an indication for sigmoidoscopy and barium enema for lower gastrointestinal malignancy in patients with chronic diarrhoea

Question 4
Concerning cohort studies, which one of the following statements is true?
A they can only be used to compare two groups with one another
B they are particularly useful with rare outcomes
C cohort studies are retrospective
D they are better than other study types for measuring the incidence of a disease in a population
E they are better than other study designs for measuring prevalence of a disease in a population

Question 5
Concerning the statistical power of studies, which one of the following statements is FALSE?
A a power calculation must always be performed before conducting randomized clinical trials
B a type II error occurs if it is claimed two treatments are the same when the study is not large enough to detect equivalence
C a type I error is where the null hypothesis is falsely rejected
D the smaller the difference you want to detect, the larger a study must be
E international journals do not publish studies that are underpowered

Question 6
Regarding crossover trial design, which one of the following statements is true?
A it can be used to compare treatments for an acute infection
B it cannot be double-blinded
C it cannot be randomised
D it is a good method for comparing analgesics in arthritis
E tends to need more patients than are required with other trial designs to get adequate statistical power

Question 7
Regarding case-control studies, which one of the following statements is FALSE?
A they are good for investigating rare diseases
B they are good for identifying rare causes of disease
C they may be uninterpretable if controls are selected poorly
D they can examine multiple risk-factors for a single disease
E they compare exposures of interest in cases and controls

Question 8
For continuous data, which one of the following statements is true?
A a positive s test (skew test) result means that the data is not normally distributed

B it is always wrong to use the mean to describe skewed data

C chi-squared is the best test for comparing skewed continuous data

D the Wilcoxon rank-sum test is best used with normally distributed data

E the interquartile range is two standard deviations wide

Question 9

The practice of evidence-based medicine (EBM) begins with the formulation of an answerable question. Which one of the following elements is NOT required for a question to be answerable?

A a particular patient or problem

B an intervention

C a comparison

D an outcome measure

E at least one relevant randomised controlled trial

Question 10

The statistical reviewer of a paper states that they are concerned that the findings are biased. In statistical terms, 'bias' means:

A there is a flaw in study design that leads to a built-in likelihood that the wrong result may be obtained

B there is a flaw in statistical analysis leading to a likelihood that the wrong result may be obtained

C there is reason to believe that the authors wanted to obtain the result that the study showed

D both study design and statistical analysis are flawed, leading to a likelihood that the wrong result may be obtained

E the study is not of sufficient statistical power to exclude the missing of a significant effect

Question 11

A researcher is trying to design a study to find out the cause (or causes) of a rare disease, about which very little is known. What study design is most likely to be appropriate?

A geographical

B cross-sectional

C cohort

D intervention

E case control

Question 12

A 95% confidence interval means:

A 95% of the data fall within the confidence interval

B there is a 95% chance that two groups are different

C that p = 0.05

D there is a 95% chance that the true value falls within the confidence interval

E there is a 95% chance that the finding is clinically significant

Question 13

Regarding the description and comparison of two groups of data, which one of the following statements is true?

A categorical data should be described as percentages and compared using a Student's t-test

B normally distributed continuous data should be described as median and range and compared using a chi-squared test

C skewed continuous data should be described as median and range and compared using a Wilcoxon rank-sum test

D normally distributed continuous data should be described as mean and standard deviation and compared using a chi-squared test

E skewed continuous data should be described as mean and standard deviation and compared using a Student's t-test

Question 14

A manuscript is submitted to a medical journal regarding a randomised trial in which a new treatment for Clostridium difficile diarrhoea is compared with an established treatment. A reviewer states that they are concerned that there might be type 2 statistical error. What does this mean? That the:

A method of statistical analysis used is inappropriate

B study has shown a difference between the treatments that is statistically significant but which is unlikely to be clinically significant

C study claims to find a difference that does not really exist, i.e. the result is a statistical fluke

D data is skewed (not normally distributed) and analysis should have used non-parametric rather than parametric statistical techniques

E study claims that there is no difference between the treatments, when in reality the trial was just too small to detect a difference

Question 15

A placebo-controlled study randomised 10 000 patients undergoing surgery for hip fracture to 160 mg aspirin / day, started preoperatively and continued for 35 days. About 1.5% of the patients allocated aspirin had DVT or pulmonary embolism (PE), compared with about 2.5% allocated placebo. Which one of the following statements about this trial is true?

A aspirin produced a 1.5% absolute risk reduction in DVT/PE

B aspirin produced a 40% absolute risk reduction in DVT/PE

C aspirin produced a 1% proportional risk reduction in DVT/PE

D aspirin produced a 40% proportional risk reduction in DVT/PE

E the Number Needed to Treat (NNT) to prevent one DVT/PE is 100/1.5 = 67

Question 16
A committee is deciding whether a trial of a new treatment against an established treatment of a malignancy is ethical. Which one of the following would mean that the trial was ethically justifiable?
A the new treatment is thought to be better than the established treatment
B the established treatment is not a very effective treatment of the malignancy
C it is not certain which of the two treatments is best
D the established treatment is effective, but has a very high incidence of significant side effects
E the malignancy is very aggressive, with a median survival of 6 months with the established treatment

Question 17
If data are skewed, then they should be summarized in the form:
A mean and standard deviation
B median and range
C mean and range
D median and standard deviation
E mean and 95% confidence intervals

Question 18
The number needed to treat (NNT) is:
A 1 divided by absolute risk reduction
B 1 divided by relative risk reduction
C 1 divided by the *p* value
D 100 divided by relative risk reduction
E the same as the absolute risk reduction

Question 19
In a study of patients with myocardial infarction, the death rate of those given aspirin is 8%, compared with 10% in those not given aspirin. This means that the:
A relative risk of death after myocardial infarction is 1.25 in those given aspirin
B relative risk reduction produced by aspirin is 2%
C number needed to treat with aspirin to prevent one death is 8
D number needed to treat with aspirin to prevent one death is 10
E absolute risk reduction produced by aspirin is 2%

Question 20
To compare two groups of categorical data, e.g. dead/alive by drug/placebo, the correct test is:
A Student's *t*-test
B Analysis of variance (ANOVA)
C Wilcoxon rank-sum
D chi-squared
E *p* value

Clinical Pharmacology

AUTHORS:
**E.H. Baker, S.F. Haydock, A.D. Hingorani,
D.J.M. Reynolds**

EDITOR:
D.J.M. Reynolds

EDITOR-IN-CHIEF:
J.D. Firth

1 Introducing clinical pharmacology

This section on clinical pharmacology gives the background to the way in which the body handles drugs (pharmacokinetics), and how drugs affect the body (pharmacodynamics). Not all effects of drugs are advantageous, and it is vitally important that all clinicians have a sound understanding of the ways in which drugs cause adverse effects and those circumstances where prescribing carries enhanced risks.

How does a prescriber decide whether to offer drug treatment in any particular condition? Which class of drugs would be most appropriate, and from within a seemingly homogeneous class of drugs which individual product should be chosen? At what dosage should it be used, by which route, which formulation, for how long? When should it be administered, will it interact with other products, what are the side effects, and what is the likely benefit that might arise from using this drug in this patient? What is the cost of the drug, does the risk–benefit seem favourable, and what does the patient think? All of these questions arise whenever we prescribe. However, even in circumstances where we might feel entirely confident, there is much to be gained from a critical analysis.

1.1 Preconceived notions versus evidence

Example 1: Which analgesic?

Case history
A patient has an inguinal hernia repair as a day case and at home that night develops pain of moderate severity. He has a choice of analgesic at home: paracetamol 1.0 g, ibuprofen 400 mg or codeine 60 mg. Which drug should he take (assuming that he can have only one) to maximize his chances of gaining an analgesic effect? (See *Pain relief and palliative care*, Sections 1.1 and 2.1.)

Clinical approach
When presented with this question I suspect that most doctors would rate these drugs in descending order of effectiveness as: codeine, ibuprofen, paracetamol. A careful meta-analysis of randomized controlled trials in acute pain has clearly shown that the rank order is ibuprofen with an NNT of 3 (number needed to treat—see *Epidemiology, statistics, clinical trials, meta-analyses and evidence-based medicine*, Section 1), followed by paracetamol 1.0 g (NNT = 4.6), with codeine 60 mg coming in a poor last with an NNT of 16. Preconceptions and medical mythology are hard to shift!

1.2 Drug interactions and safe prescribing

With so many drugs available, there are almost unlimited possibilities for drug–drug and drug–disease interactions, and it is the responsibility of every prescriber to have easy access to, and be familiar with, up-to-date information about the more common interactions and adverse effects of drugs. In the UK, the most convenient authoritative source of this information is the *British National Formulary* (BNF).

Example 2: Drug interactions can kill

Case history
A 79-year-old woman with atrial fibrillation developed a second episode of moderately severe depression and her psychiatrist prescribed a selective serotonin reuptake inhibitor (SSRI) which had helped her before. He had extensive experience in prescribing SSRIs but was unaware of a potentially significant interaction between the SSRI and the warfarin that she was taking, and did not think to check the BNF for interactions. The patient became over-anticoagulated, bled into her retroperitoneum and subsequently died. Had he checked the appendix in the BNF for interactions, the international normalized ratio (INR) could have been closely monitored, the dosage of warfarin adjusted as necessary, and the bleed and the patient's subsequent death avoided.

Develop the habit of routinely referring to the BNF for all but the most familiar prescribing decisions.

There is an ever-expanding literature on drug efficacy and safety for existing drugs, and every year around 30–40 new drugs are licensed in the UK. All prescribers must master the skills of critical appraisal, know how to access up-to-date information, and know where to receive authoritative advice and guidance. The art of good prescribing is in knowing how to apply the best available evidence to each individual patient in order to achieve the maximum benefit that they might gain, with the minimum of risk.

There are no really 'safe' biologically active drugs. There are only 'safe' physicians. (Harold A. Kaminetzky)

All of the information in this clinical pharmacology module provides a background to the therapeutics discussed in each of the specialty modules.

 Hardman JG, Limbird L, eds. *Goodman and Gilman's Pharmacological Basis of Therapeutics*, 9th edn. New York: McGraw-Hill, 1996.

McQuay HJ, Moore AJ. *An Evidence-Based Resource for Pain Relief.* Oxford: Oxford University Press, 1998.

Risk : benefit analysis of drugs in practice. *Drug Ther Bull* 1995; 33: 33–5.

2 Pharmacokinetics

2.1 Introduction

The word 'pharmacokinetics' comes from the Greek (*Pharmakon*, drug; *kineein*, to move). It literally describes the ways in which drugs move into, out of and around the body, and are handled by the tissues and organs. We use pharmacokinetics, either consciously or subconsciously, every time a prescribing decision is made, e.g. when considering how much and how often to give a drug, by what route to administer the drug, and when informing the patient how quickly it may work. Understanding of pharmacokinetics is therefore of great importance in daily clinical practice. In this section, examples of clinical problems are described and the pharmacokinetic principles required to solve these problems discussed.

2.2 Drug absorption

Example 3: Diarrhoea and the pill

Case history
A 24-year-old woman has been in hospital for 5 days with severe diarrhoea. During admission she has been taking her regular oral contraceptive pill. On discharge she asks for information about her risk of becoming pregnant.

Clinical approach
Your main concern is that her severe diarrhoea has impaired absorption of the oral contraceptive across the gastrointestinal tract, reducing plasma levels of oestrogen and progesterone and thereby increasing her chances of contraceptive failure.

Pharmacokinetics of gastrointestinal absorption

Most drug absorption in the gastrointestinal tract occurs by diffusion. For diffusion to occur, the drug must be dissolved so that individual drug molecules come into contact with the gut epithelium, and the drug must be chemically lipid soluble so that it can cross cell membranes (Fig. 1 and Table 1). Diffusion is greatest where there is the following:

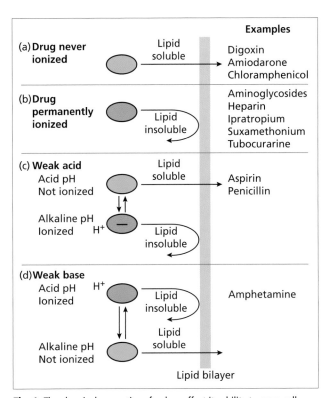

Fig. 1 The chemical properties of a drug affect its ability to cross cell membranes. (a) Drugs that are not ionized (non-polar) are lipid soluble and can cross cell membranes. (b) Ionized drugs are lipid insoluble and cannot cross cell membranes. (c, d) Many drugs are weak acids or weak bases; their lipid solubility and ability to cross cell membranes depend on the environment's pH.

• A large surface area for absorption; most drug absorption occurs in the small intestine.
• A large concentration gradient driving drug absorption from the gut lumen to the interstitium. The concentration gradient is increased by larger drug doses, which increase luminal concentration, or greater intestinal blood flow, which lowers interstitial drug concentration by removing the absorbed drug.

Other factors that affect intestinal drug absorption are shown in Table 2.

Drug preparations and absorption

Drug manufacturers alter the physical and chemical properties of drugs to control absorption characteristics (Fig. 2), e.g. nifedipine is available in a number of different preparations that are absorbed at different rates. Nifedipine capsules containing liquid are absorbed rapidly; tablets prepared for slow release of nifedipine

	Lipid soluble	Lipid insoluble
Gastrointestinal absorption	Good	Poor
Administration	Can be given orally	May need to be given parenterally
Distribution	Wide, including across blood–brain barrier and placenta	Limited, may not penetrate blood brain–barrier or cross placenta
Metabolism and elimination	Metabolism required to decrease lipid solubility before elimination	May be eliminated without metabolism
Plasma half-life	May be prolonged by 'reservoir' of drug in tissues and by requirement for metabolism	Often short, as elimination does not require metabolism

Table 1 General pharmacokinetic properties of lipid-soluble and lipid-insoluble drugs.

Properties of drug	Properties of GI tract	Interaction between drug and GI tract
Physical preparation	Site of absorption	Interaction with food or other drugs
Chemical properties	Surface area	in gut lumen, e.g.
Dose	Intestinal transit time (increased by infection, decreased by food)	• calcium, aluminium or magnesium in milk or antacids reduce tetracycline absorption
	Blood supply	• activated charcoal used to reduce absorption of drugs taken in overdose
	Enterohepatic circulation	• cholestyramine interferes with absorption of warfarin, digoxin, thyroxine
		• ingested drug altered by pH or enzymes in gut lumen, e.g. benzylpenicillin destroyed by gastric acid, insulin digested by gut enzymes

Table 2 Factors which determine drug absorption across the gastrointestinal (GI) tract.

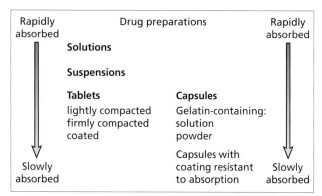

Fig. 2 Rates of absorption of oral pharmaceutical preparations.

Example 3: Diarrhoea and the pill (*continued*)

Clinical approach
Severe diarrhoea causes decreased intestinal transit time. In our patient on the oral contraceptive pill, this would have reduced contact of ingested hormones with the intestinal epithelium and thus reduced absorption of oestrogen and progesterone. Severe diarrhoea may also disrupt the enterohepatic circulation, which maintains plasma concentrations of ethinyloestradiol (Fig. 3 and Table 3). A fall in the plasma levels of oestrogen and progesterone increases the chance of ovulation and conception.

Armed with this pharmacokinetic knowledge you should advise your patient:
• to continue the oral contraceptive pill, but use other contra-ceptive methods until she is well, and for 7 days after recovery
• that the diarrhoea is more likely to have reduced her contraceptive protection if she is at the beginning or end of her pill cycle. At these times, reduced hormone absorption will extend the duration of low plasma hormone levels and protection against pregnancy is reduced. She should therefore omit the 7-day pill-free interval if she is at the end of a cycle.

and long-acting tablets with absorption-resistant coating are absorbed more slowly. Other drug preparations are designed to release the drug at a specific site in the gastrointestinal tract where its actions are required, e.g. sulfasalazine (sulphasalazine), used to maintain remission in ulcerative colitis, consists of sulphapyridine and 5-aminosalicylic acid joined by an azo bond. This complex passes unchanged through the gastrointestinal tract until it reaches the large intestine, where colonic bacteria split the azo bond and release the 5-aminosalicylic acid to act on the colon.

Routes of drug administration

In general, the oral route is used for drug administration because it is acceptable and convenient for the patient. However, other routes of administration (Table 4) may be necessary or preferable for drugs that:

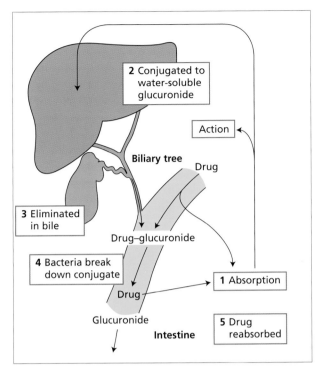

Fig. 3 The enterohepatic circulation. Absorbed drugs (step 1) are modified by conjugation, e.g. with glucuronate to increase water solubility (step 2) and are excreted in the bile (step 3). Once in the gut, bacteria act to break up the drug–glucuronide conjugate (step 4). If the released unconjugated drug is lipid soluble, it will be reabsorbed in the gastrointestinal tract (step 5). This 'enterohepatic circulation' of drugs can form a circulating reservoir of up to 20% of the total concentration of drug in the body. The enterohepatic circulation is interrupted by antibiotics that alter gut flora, e.g. neomycin, and less so by severe diarrhoea.

Table 3 Drugs recycled by the enterohepatic circulation.

Ethinyloestriadiol (in many oral contraceptives)
Sulindac (NSAID)
Pentaerythritol tetranitrate (oral nitrate)
Digoxin
Morphine
Chloramphenicol
Vecuronium (muscle relaxant)
Rifampicin

- are not absorbed when given orally
- are irritant to the gastrointestinal tract
- cause side effects when given orally, which can be avoided by topical administration
- act too slowly or unpredictably when given orally
- undergo extensive (Table 5) or unpredictable pre-systemic metabolism.

Non-oral routes of drug administration and some of their advantages and disadvantages are shown in Table 4.

Bioavailability

A drug exerts its action once it has reached the circulation and gained access to tissues and receptors. Drugs injected directly into a vein are 100% bioavailable. Drugs given orally are less than 100% bioavailable because the drug may be incompletely absorbed, or it may undergo pre-systemic metabolism by drug-metabolizing enzymes in the gut wall or liver before reaching the circulation.

Table 4 Alternative routes of drug administration—their uses and problems.

	Route	Use	Potential problems
GI tract	Buccal Sublingual Rectal	Drugs requiring quick action, e.g. aspirin during MI, GTN for angina. Where drugs cannot be swallowed but do not need to be injected, e.g. sublingual buprenorphine analgesia or rectal metronidazole after GI surgery	Rectal administration may be unacceptable. Many drugs are not absorbed sufficiently by these routes
Injection (parenteral)	Intravenous Intramuscular Subcutaneous Intradermal Into body cavity or tissue	Where drugs cannot be absorbed or are destroyed in the GI tract (see Table 1). Where swift onset or termination of drug action is required	Injection may be painful and unacceptable to patient. Requires help or training by health-care professional. May introduce infection
Topical	ENT Eye Skin Inhaled	For local use: Administered directly to site of action. Reduces systemic side effects of drug, e.g. inhaled vs oral steroids for asthma. For systemic use: Alternative routes where GI administration is not possible which avoids injections, e.g. intranasal vasopressin	May get local allergy. Despite local administration systemic effects may occur, e.g. side effects of β blockers given into the eye for glaucoma

ENT, ear, nose and throat; GI, gastrointestinal; GTN, glyceryl trinitrate; MI, myocardial infarction.

Table 5 Example of oral and parenteral doses of drugs undergoing extensive presystemic (first-pass) metabolism.

Drug undergoing extensive presystemic metabolism	Oral dose (mg)	Comparable intravenous dose
Metoprolol	50–100	5–15 mg
Atenolol	50–100	2.5–10 mg
Verapamil	40–120	5–10 mg
Salbutamol	4	250 mcg

Where a drug undergoes extensive presystemic metabolism, the intravenous dose required to achieve a given plasma level and have a therapeutic effect is lower than the oral dose required to have the same effect (Table 5). It is particularly important to check the dose of drugs that can be given both orally and intravenously before administration by either route.

Rowland M, Tozer TN. *Clinical Pharmacokinetics: Concepts and Applications*, 3rd edn. Lippincott, Williams and Wilkins, 1995.

2.3 Drug distribution

Example 4: Sinemet and variation of drug distribution

Case history
A 73-year-old man with Parkinson's disease is commenced on Sinemet (levodopa with carbidopa). After 1 week he is considerably more mobile, but has developed nausea and vomiting. (See *Neurology*, Sections 1.3 and 2.3.)

Clinical approach
Loss of dopaminergic neurons in the extrapyramidal system results in abnormal movement control with hypokinesia, rigidity and tremor—the symptoms of Parkinson's disease.

These symptoms can be relieved by augmenting the effects of dopamine, using the precursor, levodopa, which is converted by dopa decarboxylase to dopamine in the brain. However, levodopa is also metabolized to dopamine in the periphery and causes side effects, including nausea and vomiting, through the action of dopamine at the area postrema in the brain stem (site of the chemoreceptor trigger zone for emesis), which has a deficient blood–brain barrier. Co-administration of carbidopa, a dopa decarboxylase inhibitor, prevents levodopa metabolism and side effects in the periphery, including the area postrema; however, as it does not cross the blood–brain barrier, carbidopa does not affect the central conversion of levodopa to dopamine. The success of treatment regimens for Parkinson's disease is dependent on the different distribution properties of the drugs that are used.

Body water compartments

Fig. 4 Distribution of drugs in the body. Lipid-insoluble drugs remain in the extracellular water because they cannot cross cell membranes. Lipid-soluble drugs may cross freely into all body water compartments. Drugs that are extensively bound to plasma proteins stay mostly in the plasma, even if lipid soluble. Tissue-bound drugs form a drug reservoir in the tissues. CSF, cerebrospinal fluid.

Pharmacokinetics of drug distribution

Distribution of individual drugs into different body compartments depends on (Fig. 4):
- the lipid solubility of the drug
- binding of the drug to plasma and tissue proteins.

Lipid solubility and drug distribution

Lipid-insoluble drugs remain largely in the extracellular water. Lipid-soluble drugs distribute freely throughout the body and cross into transcellular compartments such as the cerebrospinal fluid (CSF). Many lipid-soluble drugs are stored in physical solution in fat (see Fig. 1 and Table 1).

The lipid solubility of drugs that are weak acids or weak bases will change depending on the pH of the body compartment that they are in, e.g. a weak acid such as aspirin (salicylic acid) will be un-ionized and lipid soluble at low pH in the stomach and hence freely absorbed. However, once in intestinal cells that have an intracellular pH of 7.35–7.45, the salicylic acid becomes ionized and is less able to move out of the cell. This process is known as pH partitioning.

Plasma protein and tissue binding

Some drugs bind extensively to plasma proteins and so remain largely in the plasma. Other drugs are extensively bound to tissue sites, usually proteins, phospholipids or nucleoproteins, and so accumulate in tissues (Table 6).

Table 6 Examples of drugs which bind to plasma and tissue proteins or form a reservoir in lipids.

Reservoir site	Drug
Plasma proteins	
Albumin	Warfarin, diazepam, frusemide, tolbutamide, clofibrate, phenytoin, amitryptiline
Lipoprotein, α-acid glycoprotein	Basic drugs (e.g. quinidine, chlorpromazine, imipramine).
Other sites	
Tissue sites	Amiodarone, chloroquine, digoxin
Lipid stores	Benzodiazepines, verapamil, lignocaine

Clinical significance of drug distribution

Drug action

For a drug to have a biological effect, first it has to reach the target site of action. Lipid-insoluble drugs distribute poorly and may not reach this target site, e.g. lipid-insoluble aminoglycoside antibiotics are not generally used for meningitis because they transfer poorly into the CSF, even where the blood–brain barrier is damaged by inflammation.

Loading dose

Drugs that are lipid soluble, or protein or tissue bound, distribute widely. When treatment with such drugs is started, it takes some time for lipid- or drug-binding sites to become saturated and for plasma concentrations to rise to therapeutic levels. When it is important to achieve therapeutic plasma concentrations quickly, a large first dose (loading dose) is given to saturate the lipid or binding sites of the drug rapidly.

Drug reservoirs

Once the distribution sites of a lipid-soluble or protein- or tissue-bound drug have been saturated, the plasma concentration of the drug reaches a steady state. When administration of the drug is discontinued and the plasma concentration starts to fall through the effects of drug metabolism and excretion, the drug redistributes into plasma from lipid or tissue reservoirs, maintaining the plasma concentration. It is important to remember that the effects of such drugs may take some time to wear off, and there is potential for side effects or drug interactions for days or weeks after stopping the drug.

Drug interactions

Where two drugs that bind to the same binding site (e.g.

Example 4: Sinemet and variation of drug distribution (*continued*)

Clinical approach
Peripheral conversion of levodopa to dopamine stimulates dopamine (D_2) receptors in the chemoreceptor trigger zone in the brain stem, triggering the troublesome side effects of nausea and vomiting. Co-administration of carbidopa reduces the incidence of nausea and vomiting in patients taking levodopa from 80% to 15%, by inhibiting peripheral levodopa metabolism. Your patient, who is still suffering from nausea and vomiting despite taking carbidopa, can be helped by the antiemetic domperidone. Domperidone inhibits the emetic action of dopamine by blocking D_2-receptors in the chemo-receptor trigger zone, but it does not interfere with the central therapeutic actions of levodopa because, like carbidopa, it does not cross the blood–brain barrier to a significant degree.

plasma proteins) are given together, binding of one or other drug may be reduced. The plasma concentration of the displaced drug may therefore rise, increasing the risk of drug toxicity. In practice, however, drug interactions at binding sites rarely have clinical significance.

2.4 Drug metabolism

The body 'sees' drugs as 'foreign' and attempts to expel them by metabolism and elimination. Most of these processes occur in the liver and kidneys, although other tissues and organs may play an additional role. A general principle is that drugs that are lipid soluble are difficult to excrete, because when they enter the urine or bile they are reabsorbed across cell membranes back into the body. Removal of lipid-soluble drugs from the body thus requires metabolism to make them more water soluble, followed by elimination of the metabolites in the urine or bile. Drugs that are already water soluble can be excreted without metabolism.

Example 5: Paracetamol overdose

Case history
A 17-year-old woman is admitted having taken 30 paracetamol tablets 1 h previously. She now regrets this and denies suicidal intent. (See *Emergency medicine*, Section 2.1.)

Clinical approach
Your main concern is that this paracetamol overdose will lead to liver damage if untreated.

Prevention of liver damage depends on reducing the amount of *N*-acetyl-*p*-benzoquinone imine (NABQI) available to cause hepatic necrosis. This can be done by reducing paracetamol absorption and by increasing the conjugation of NABQI.

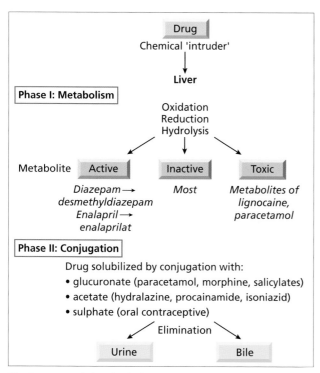

Fig. 5 Drug metabolism by the liver.

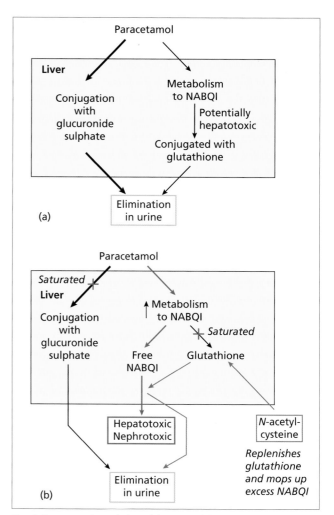

Fig. 6 Paracetamol metabolism: (a) at normal dose; (b) after paracetamol overdose and *N*-acetylcysteine treatment. NABQI, *N*-acetyl-*p*-benzoquinone imine.

Paracetamol pharmacokinetics

Drugs are metabolized by the liver in two phases (Fig. 5); the metabolism of paracetamol illustrates this well (Fig. 6). At recommended daily doses (maximum 4 g, i.e. 8 × 500 mg tablets over 24 h), most of the paracetamol is inactivated by conjugation with glucuronide or sulphate (phase II metabolism). A small amount of paracetamol is oxidized by cytochrome P450 enzymes to the reactive metabolite *N*-acetyl-*p*-benzoquinone imine (NABQI) (phase I metabolism). NABQI can cause cell damage, both by forming covalent bonds with cell constituents, such as key enzymes, and by generation of oxygen radicals that are cytotoxic. However, glutathione protects cells from damage by NABQI by both mopping up toxic oxygen radicals and conjugating NABQI (phase II metabolism). Both paracetamol and NABQI are made water soluble by conjugation and can be excreted in the urine.

In overdose, mechanisms that conjugate paracetamol to glucuronide or sulphate become saturated and metabolism of paracetamol to NABQI is increased (see Fig. 6). When the amount of NABQI formed is greater than the glutathione available, cell damage occurs and, as most paracetamol metabolism occurs in the liver, hepatic necrosis and hepatic failure occur. Cytochrome P450 enzymes are also present in the kidney, where generation of NABQI can result in acute tubular necrosis and renal failure.

Reducing paracetamol absorption

If paracetamol absorption is reduced, less NABQI will be generated. As this patient has presented early (1 h after taking the overdose), paracetamol absorption might be reduced by oral activated charcoal. Gastric lavage may have a place in patients who have taken a large, potentially life-threatening overdose, if performed within 60 min of ingestion, but there is no convincing evidence from randomized clinical trials for the effectiveness of either gastric lavage or activated charcoal in paracetamol poisoning.

Increasing conjugation of NABQI

The aim of treatment is to increase glutathione levels so that toxic NABQI can be conjugated. Glutathione itself cannot be given because it penetrates cells poorly. *N*-acetylcysteine, which enters cells and is metabolized to glutathione, is given intravenously. (See *Emergency medicine*, Section 2.1.)

Drug-metabolizing enzymes

Enzymes that metabolize drugs are found primarily in the smooth endoplasmic reticulum of liver cells, but are also in cells of the kidney, lung and intestinal epithelium, and in the plasma. There are many different types of drug-metabolizing enzymes, which can be divided into those that catalyse phase I and those that catalyse phase II reactions (see Fig. 5).

Phase I reactions

Phase I reactions make the substrate drug more polar (less lipid soluble) and may create a 'reactive' site that is susceptible to conjugation (phase II reactions). Drugs may be inactivated by phase I reactions, although they may also be activated or converted to toxic metabolites (see Fig. 5). Prodrugs are inactive drugs requiring conversion to an active form by metabolism before they can exert a therapeutic effect (Table 7). Phase I reactions include the following:

• Oxidation (loss of electrons): this is catalysed by, for example, cytochrome P450 enzymes, oxidases, alcohol and aldehyde dehydrogenases.

• Reduction (gain of electrons): these reactions are uncommon but include metabolism of warfarin by ketoreductase.

• Hydrolysis: catalysed insertion of a H_2O molecule into a drug, e.g. by esterases, proteases, peptidases. These reactions occur predominantly in the plasma.

Table 7 Prodrugs which require activation by the liver to exert an effect.

Prodrug	Active metabolite
Enalapril	Enalaprilat
Cyclophosphamide	Phosphoramide mustard
Azathioprine	Mercaptopurine
Zidovudine	Zidovudine triphosphate
Cortisone	Hydrocortisone
Chloral hydrate	Trichloroethanol

The cytochrome P450 enzyme family

The cytochrome P450 enzyme family (CYP) is responsible for most phase I drug metabolism. There are many different CYP isoenzymes, which are grouped into families and subfamilies defined by their molecular structure, e.g. CYP 1A2 is a member of family 1 and subfamily A. Each isoenzyme metabolizes specific substrates, although the actions of different isoenzymes may overlap. The existence of a large number of CYP isoenzymes allows the body to detoxify and excrete a wide range of exogenous compounds, as well as adapting easily to metabolize new substances. The rate of drug metabolism by CYP isoenzymes depends on genetic and environmental factors.

Table 8 Genetic variants of drug-metabolizing enzymes.

	Enzyme	Commonly used drugs metabolized by enzyme	Genetic variants affecting drug metabolism
Phase I reactions	CYP 2C8	Diazepam Omeprazole Barbiturates	Poor metabolizers of the CYP 2C subfamily: 20−25% Asians
	CYP 2C18/19	Tricyclic antidepressants Diazepam Mephenytoin Omeprazole Oxicam drugs Proguanil Propranolol	Poor metabolizers: 18% Japanese 19% African Americans 8% Africans 3−5% Caucasians
	CYP 2D6	β blockers Tricyclic antidepressants SSRIs MAO-I (amiflavine) Many typical and atypical antipsychotics Many antiarrhythmics (Dihydro)codeine Ecstasy Ondansetron	Poor metabolizers: 5−10% Caucasians
Phase II reactions	Acetylating enzyme	Isoniazid Hydralazine Dapsone Sulphasalazine Procainamide	Rapid acetylators: 88% Japanese 52% African Americans 48% White Americans Approx. 35% North Europeans

MAO-I, monoamine oxidase inhibitor; SSRIs, selective serotonin reuptake inhibitors.

GENETIC FACTORS

Genetic variants of cytochrome P450 isoenzymes metabolize drugs at different rates (Table 8). 'Poor metabolizers', who metabolize drugs slowly, may be particularly susceptible to the accumulation of a drug in the body and hence to side effects. 'Rapid metabolizers', who are able to clear a drug quickly, may avoid side effects but may require larger doses of the drug to achieve the desired clinical effect.

ENVIRONMENTAL FACTORS

Where exposure to 'foreign' substances such as drugs, dietary components or pollutants is increased, CYP enzyme activity is induced (increased) to increase clearance of the substance. Conversely, CYP enzyme activity can be inhibited by drugs or dietary constituents.

 Dietary components that affect liver enzyme activity may interact with drugs metabolized by liver enzymes, e.g. constituents of grapefruit juice inhibit CYP 3A4. If patients taking drugs metabolized by CYP 3A4 (e.g. terfenadine) drink grapefruit juice, plasma levels of the ingested drug increase and the risk of toxic effects (prolonged QT and dysrhythmias with terfenadine) increases.

Phase II reactions

Phase II reactions catalyse coupling of a drug or polar metabolite to a substrate molecule. Conjugated drugs are inert and water soluble, and are eliminated in the urine or bile. Drugs may be conjugated with:
• glucuronate (catalysed by glucuronyl transferase)
• acetate from acetyl-CoA (catalysed by *N*-acetyltransferases)
• sulphate
• amino acids
• glutathione.

Genetic variants of conjugating enzymes, particularly *N*-acetyltransferases, may influence the rate of conjugating reactions (see Table 8). Consider, for instance, the use of isoniazid in the treatment of tuberculosis. Isoniazid is metabolized by acetylation and excreted in the urine, its metabolites being potentially hepatotoxic. Fast acetylators, who conjugate and clear isoniazid quickly, may require increased doses for eradication of tuberculosis but are at risk of hepatotoxicity from isoniazid metabolites. Slow acetylators, who clear isoniazid more slowly, are at risk of isoniazid accumulation with peripheral neuropathy. Consider also that slow acetylators taking hydralazine or procainamide are at risk of developing antinuclear antibodies that cause a form of systemic lupus erythematosus. (See *Rheumatology and clinical immunology*, Sections 2.4.1 and 3.2.)

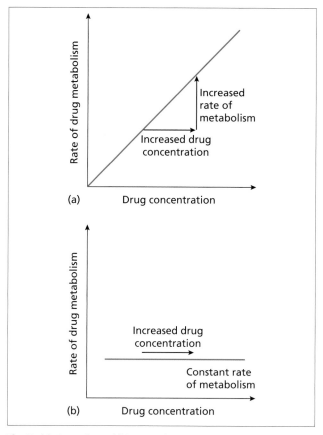

Fig. 7 (a) First-order and (b) zero-order kinetics.

Time course of drug metabolism by enzymes

First-order metabolism

The rate of drug metabolism by most drug-metabolizing enzymes increases in direct proportion to the concentration of drug available. Thus a constant fraction of the drug available will be processed (Fig. 7). Increasing or decreasing the dose of a drug metabolized by first-order processes will result in a predictable change in plasma concentration.

Zero-order metabolism

Some drug-metabolizing enzymes become saturated as the concentration of the drug increases. Once this saturation point has been reached, the enzyme can metabolize a constant amount of the drug, but a further increase in the available drug does not result in increased processing of the drug (Fig. 7). When a drug is metabolized by a zero-order process, a dose increase will result in a large and disproportionate increase in plasma concentration, which has the potential to produce toxicity. Removal of excessive drug from the body, e.g. after an overdose, is also slow where metabolism is by zero-order processes. The main examples of drugs metabolized by zero-order processes are ethanol and phenytoin.

Time course of other pharmacokinetic processes

Other pharmacokinetic processes, including absorption, distribution and elimination, may exhibit either zero- or first-order kinetics, e.g. drug absorption across cell membranes by transport proteins could be a first-order process if absorption increases with increased drug concentration, or a zero-order process if drug transfer by the transport protein becomes saturated.

Cytochrome P450 enzymes and drug interactions (Table 9)

Example 6: An interaction leading to theophylline toxicity

Case history
A 65-year-old man, taking theophylline for chronic obstructive pulmonary disease, is admitted with convulsions. He has recently started taking ciprofloxacin for a chest infection. (See *Respiratory medicine*, Section 1.3 and *Emergency medicine*, Section 1.10.)

Clinical approach
You are concerned that the convulsions in this patient are caused by theophylline toxicity, precipitated by concurrent therapy with ciprofloxacin.

Enzyme inhibition

Theophylline is cleared from the body by CYP 1A2 metabolism followed by conjugation and elimination. Ciprofloxacin inhibits the actions of CYP 1A2 so, if a patient who is already receiving theophylline starts taking ciprofloxacin, theophylline metabolism will be reduced and theophylline plasma concentrations will rise—an interaction that is clinically significant because theophylline has a narrow therapeutic range (Fig. 8). This means that the plasma concentration of theophylline having a therapeutic effect is only slightly lower than the theophylline concentration that will cause toxic effects such as nausea, irritability, dysrhythmias and convulsions. Thus, a relatively small decrease in theophylline metabolism will cause an increase in theophylline concentration sufficient to cause toxicity. In addition to its effect on theophylline metabolism, ciprofloxacin may also independently lower seizure thresholds, thereby further increasing the likelihood of seizure in this patient.

Other substrates for liver enzymes that have a narrow therapeutic range are shown in Table 9. Note also that, in some cases, the presence of the disease process narrows the therapeutic window.

Table 9 Drug interactions and the cytochrome P450 system.

CYP450 substrates with narrow therapeutic range	Drugs that inhibit CYP450 enzymes	Drugs that induce CYP450 enzymes
Warfarin	Cimetidine	Phenytoin
Theophylline	Ciprofloxacin	Phenobarbitone
Cyclosporin	Erythromycin	Carbamazepine
Ethinyloestradiol	Sodium valproate	Rifampicin
Phenytoin	Isoniazid	Griseofulvin
		Alcohol
		Tobacco smoke
		Primidone
		Sulphinpyrazone
		Meprobamate
		Glutethimide

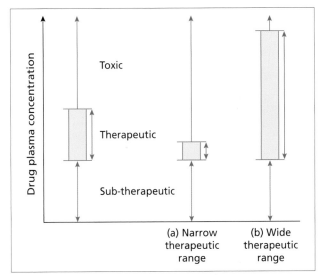

Fig. 8 Therapeutic range: the therapeutic range describes plasma concentrations at which a drug exerts a safe therapeutic effect. (a) Where the range is narrow, therapeutic plasma concentrations are close to toxic plasma concentrations, and a small change in dose or drug metabolism may precipitate drug toxicity. (b) Where the range is wide, therapeutic plasma concentrations are much lower than toxic concentrations, and toxicity is unlikely.

Theophylline toxicity may be precipitated by co-administration of ciprofloxacin or erythromycin, both of which inhibit liver enzyme activity and reduce theophylline metabolism.

Enzyme induction

Drugs that induce liver enzymes increase the metabolism of drugs that are substrates for the same enzymes (Table 9), causing a fall in plasma concentration of the substrate drug that may reduce the therapeutic effect of that drug.

A classic example of this type of drug interaction is seen where rifampicin and the combined oral contraceptive pill are co-administered. Rifampicin induces CYP enzymes that metabolize oestrogen, resulting in a fall in plasma oestrogen levels and loss of contraceptive effect.

Example 6: An interaction leading to theophylline toxicity (*continued*)

Clinical approach
In this patient, theophylline toxicity could have been prevented if he had been given a different antibiotic instead of the ciprofloxacin, e.g. amoxycillin, which does not inhibit liver enzymes. If treatment with ciprofloxacin or erythromycin, which also inhibits liver enzymes, was unavoidable, then a reduction in theophylline dosage should have been considered during antibiotic treatment.

Meyer UA, Zanger UM. Molecular mechanisms of genetic polymorphisms of drug metabolism. *Annu Rev Pharmacol Toxicol* 1997; 37: 269–96.
Tanaka E. Update: genetic polymorphism of drug metabolizing enzymes in humans. *J Clin Pharmacol Ther* 1999; 24: 323–9.
Vale JA. Position statement: gastric lavage. American Academy of Clinical Toxicology; European Association of Poisons Centres and Clinical Toxicologists. *J Toxicol Clin Toxicol* 1997; 35: 711–19.
Vale JA, Proudfoot A. Paracetamol. *Medicine* 1999; 27: 50–2.

2.5 Drug elimination

Example 7: Slowing drug elimination can make treatment simpler

Case history
A 22-year-old man of no fixed abode attends a walk-in genitourinary clinic complaining of dysuria and urethral discharge. He requires treatment for gonorrhoea. (See *Infectious diseases*, Section 1.32.)

Clinical approach
Your main concern is to ensure treatment for his gonorrhoea to:
• prevent worsening illness
• prevent spread to sexual contacts.
You wish to give him a course of amoxycillin. However, given his social circumstances, you are concerned that he may have problems following a treatment regimen or attending for follow-up.

Table 10 Routes of drug elimination.

Excretion route	Comment
Urine	Most drugs
Faeces	Biliary excretion (see Table 3)
	Unabsorbed drug passes out in faeces
Lung	Exhaled drugs, e.g. volatile anaesthetics, ethanol, paraldehyde
Breast milk	A small amount of most drugs appears in breast milk, but contributes little to elimination

Pharmacokinetics of drug elimination

Drugs are eliminated from the body by a number of routes (Table 10). To be eliminated by the kidney the drug must pass into the urine (Fig. 9). This takes place by:
• glomerular filtration (drugs of molecular weight <20 000)
• active transport by cation or anion transporters, which pump the drug into the urine across the renal tubular epithelium.

In addition, drugs must be lipid insoluble to remain in the urine and not be reabsorbed in the renal tubule.

Clearance

Renal clearance is defined as the volume of plasma that contains the amount of drug cleared out of the body in a unit of time. This depends on the glomerular filtration rate (GFR) and the mechanisms of transport of the drug into and out of the renal tubule. Examples are shown below.

Gallamine

Gallamine is a non-depolarizing neuromuscular blocking agent (muscle relaxant), now rarely used. It is still notable because it enters the urine by glomerular filtration, but it is not reabsorbed or secreted in the renal tubules. Hence the renal clearance of gallamine will be the same as the GFR. If the GFR is 120 mL/min, then 120 mL of plasma will be completely cleared of gallamine every minute.

Penicillin

Approximately 20% of the penicillin delivered to the glomeruli is filtered into the urine. The other 80% remains in the plasma and passes in the efferent arterioles to the renal tubules. Anion transporters in the renal tubules actively secrete this penicillin into the urine. The blood passing through the kidney is thus almost

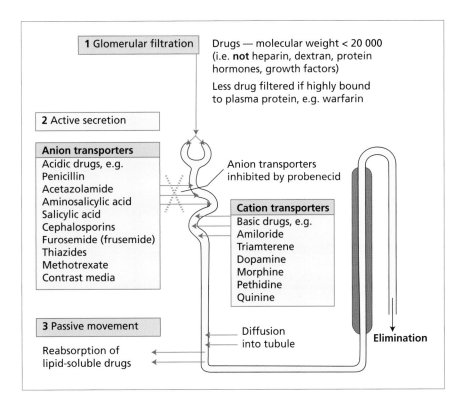

Fig. 9 Mechanisms of renal drug elimination.

completely cleared of penicillin and the renal clearance is much greater than the GFR. Approximately 480 mL plasma are cleared of penicillin every minute.

Diazepam

Diazepam is lipid soluble, thus most of the diazepam excreted into the urine is reabsorbed back into the blood. Excretion of diazepam is very slow and clearance is much less than the GFR.

Example 7: Slowing drug elimination can make treatment simpler *(continued)*

Clinical approach
Amoxycillin is commonly effective against gonorrhoea and could be useful in this patient. However, as amoxycillin is actively secreted into the renal tubule by anion exchangers, its renal clearance is extremely rapid and it has a half-life ($t_{1/2}$) of less than 2 h. Amoxycillin alone is therefore not ideal as a single-dose treatment to eradicate the gonococci. The renal clearance of amoxycillin can be reduced by giving amoxycillin with probenecid. Probenecid competes for the anion transporter, reducing secretion of amoxycillin into the renal tubule and increasing its duration of action. A single dose of amoxycillin 3 g with probenecid 1 g has been shown to cure over 98% of men with uncomplicated gonococcal urethritis. Probenecid also delays excretion and prolongs the action of other drugs secreted by the anion transporter (e.g. cephalosporins).

2.6 Plasma half-life and steady-state plasma concentrations

Example 8: A side effect of digoxin

Case history
A 72-year-old man taking digoxin 250 µg daily for atrial fibrillation complains of nausea, attributed to mild digoxin excess. The dose of digoxin is reduced to 125 µg daily, but the next day his nausea persists. (See *Cardiology*, Sections 1.1 and 1.6.)

Clinical approach
Adjustment of his digoxin dose requires knowledge of pharmacokinetic principles.

Pharmacokinetics

Plasma concentration

As soon as a drug is absorbed into the plasma, removal from the plasma commences, the plasma concentration of the drug being the sum of the processes of absorption, distribution, metabolism and elimination. The plasma concentration of a drug is important because this is the major determinant of the concentration of a drug at the target site.

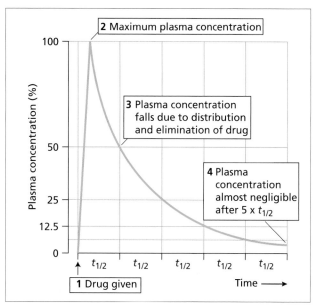

Fig. 10 Plasma half-life ($t_{1/2}$) of a drug: plasma concentration after a single dose.

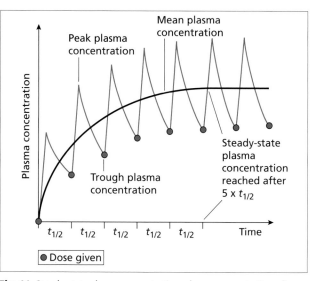

Fig. 11 Steady-state plasma concentration: plasma concentration after repeated dosing.

Half-life

The plasma half-life ($t_{1/2}$) of a drug is defined as the time taken for the plasma concentration of a drug to fall by half. Drugs that are removed from the plasma rapidly have a short half-life, e.g. amoxycillin is rapidly cleared by the renal tubules and has a half-life of about 2 h. Drugs that are removed from the plasma slowly have a long half-life, e.g. diazepam is slowly eliminated by the kidney and has a $t_{1/2}$ of about 40 h.

Steady-state plasma concentrations

After the first dose of a drug is given and absorbed, it is removed from the plasma almost completely over a time equivalent to four to five half-lives of that drug (Fig. 10). Where repeat doses of the drug are given, the average plasma concentration of the drug increases until drug absorption and removal are in equilibrium and a steady-state plasma concentration is reached. Where a consistent dosing regimen is used, steady-state plasma concentrations will be achieved after five half-lives of the drug (Fig. 11).

Drug dose and dose interval

For a given dosing regimen it will always take five half-lives of the drug to reach a steady-state plasma concentration of that drug. However, the level of the steady-state plasma concentration will be determined by the dosage of the drug, and the magnitude of swings in plasma concentration around the steady-state concentration will be determined by the dosing interval.

Example 8: A side effect of digoxin (continued)

Clinical approach
Digoxin has a $t_{1/2}$ of around 36 h. It will take approximately 7.5 days (5 × $t_{1/2}$) for the plasma concentration of digoxin in your patient to fall to a new steady-state level after this dose reduction. You would therefore expect his symptoms to resolve over several days.

2.7 Drug monitoring

Example 8: A side effect of digoxin (continued)

Case history
At a follow-up appointment 3 weeks later, the patient continues to complain of nausea and also is having frequent nose bleeds. On questioning, he is unclear which tablets he is taking, but has packets of tablets containing digoxin 250 µg and warfarin 5 mg.

Clinical approach
Your main concerns are:
• his nausea may be caused by digoxin toxicity
• his nose bleeds may indicate excessive anticoagulation by warfarin.
You need to check these suspicions by drug monitoring.

Monitoring drug therapy

Every patient who takes any medication should be 'monitored' for:
• drug effectiveness
• drug toxicity.

Table 11 Drugs commonly monitored by plasma concentration measurement.

Drug	$t_{1/2}$ (h)	Purpose of monitoring	Timing of measurement	Time to steady state
Digoxin	36	Therapeutic? Toxic?	At least 6 h after dose or immediately predose	7 days (longer in renal failure)
Lithium	22 (±8)	Therapeutic? Toxic?	12 h after dose	3–7 days
Phenytoin	6–24	Therapeutic? Toxic?	Immediately prior to next dose	7 days or longer (variable)
Aminoglycosides, e.g. gentamicin (given i.v. tds)	2–3	Therapeutic? Toxic?	Trough—immediately prior to next dose Peak—30 min post dose	12–40 h (longer in renal failure)

Monitoring can be done by the following:
• Subjective reporting by the patient, e.g. relief of symptoms, complaints of side effects.
• Measurement of the effects of a drug (pharmacodynamic monitoring), e.g. blood pressure in patients taking antihypertensives, plasma cholesterol concentration in a patient taking a statin, INR measurement in a patient taking warfarin.
• Measurement of plasma concentration of drug (pharmacokinetic monitoring).

Drug plasma concentration measurement

The monitoring of drug concentration in plasma is only useful under the following circumstances:
• The drug concentration can be measured accurately and there are no significant pharmacologically active metabolites that are not measured.
• The plasma concentration reflects drug action, i.e. a therapeutic range can be defined below which levels are likely to be subtherapeutic and above which drug levels are likely to have toxic effects (see Fig. 8).
• The therapeutic or toxic effects of the drug cannot be measured more simply and reliably by clinical measurements (as above).

Drug concentrations vary in the plasma between doses, being lowest just before a dose and highest shortly after a dose. Timing of sampling for measurement of plasma concentration must be considered carefully in the interpretation of plasma drug levels. Examples of drugs that are commonly monitored by measuring plasma concentrations are shown in Table 11.

Example 8: A side effect of digoxin (continued)

Clinical approach
Digoxin. Measurement of plasma digoxin concentration will be useful in this patient to determine whether his nausea is caused by digoxin toxicity. Where the dosing regimen is known, sampling for measurement of digoxin concentration should be done between 6 and 18 h after the last dose. The measured concentration can then be compared against values that define therapeutic and toxic levels. In this patient, a 'random' digoxin level should be measured because the time of the last dose is not known. Note also that it is very important to take blood for a potassium concentration at the same time as the digoxin concentration is measured, because it is possible to have digoxin toxicity with a digoxin concentration within the notional therapeutic range when there is coexistent hypokalaemia.
Warfarin. Nose bleeds in a patient on warfarin may be caused by excessive anticoagulation. Direct measurement of the effect of warfarin using the INR is more useful than trying to measure warfarin plasma levels.

Aronson JK, Hardman M, Reynolds DJM. *ABC of Monitoring Drug Therapy.* London: BMJ Publishing Group, 1993.

③ Pharmacodynamics

This aspect of clinical pharmacology is concerned with how drugs exert their effects on the body. An understanding of the mechanism of drug action provides insights into expected benefits and adverse effects, and whether a drug is likely to enhance or limit the action of a second agent. This understanding can also allow prediction of the likely effects of a disease process on the response to a drug, and how a drug's action might be altered as a result of changes in normal physiology, e.g. during pregnancy or at the extremes of age.

 In the past, the therapeutic properties of compounds were identified empirically. Examples include aspirin, digoxin and glyceryl trinitrate. Today, a more systematic approach to drug design is taken. Studies of physiology and pathophysiology are used to identify new therapeutic targets for which novel compounds are then synthesized (Table 12).

3.1 How drugs exert their effects

Most drugs act by binding to proteins in the body, thereby activating, inhibiting or in some way modifying their normal function (Fig. 12 and Table 13). The most important classes of drug target are:
• membrane or cytoplasmic receptors for endogenous signalling molecules, such as hormones and neurotransmitters
• enzymes
• ion channels
• transporters of small molecules, such as amino acids.

Table 12 Newly introduced drugs targeting novel targets.

Drug	Target	Use
Sildenafil	Phosphodiesterase type V	Erectile impotence
abciximab	Platelet glycoprotein IIb/IIIa receptor	Inhibition of thrombosis following coronary stent insertion
Simvastatin	HMG-CoA reductase	Hypercholesterolaemia
Montelukast	Cysteinyl leukotriene receptor	Asthma
Losartan	Angiotensin II receptor	Hypertension, heart failure

HMG, hydroxymethylglutaryl.

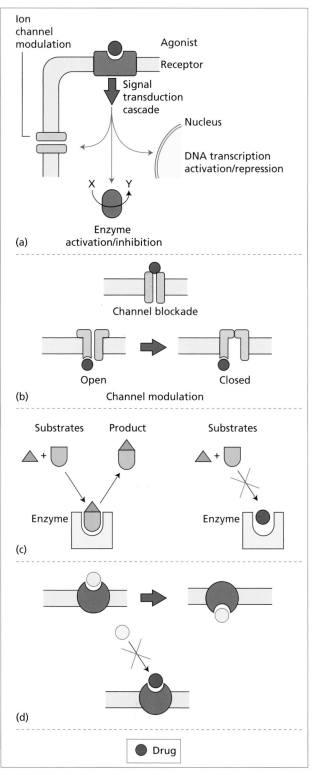

Fig. 12 Molecular targets for drugs. The major targets for drugs are cellular proteins which include (a) membrane receptors, (b) ion channels, (c) enzymes and (d) transporters.

52

Table 13 Targets for some commonly used drugs.

	Target	Drug	
		Agonist	Antagonist
Receptor	ACh nicotinic (ganglionic)	—	Trimetaphan
	ACh nicotinic (NMJ)	Suxamethonium	D-Tubocurarine
	ACh muscarinic	Pilocarpine	Atropine, ipratropium, hyoscine, orphenadrine
	α_1-Adrenoceptor	Norepinephrine (noradrenaline)	Phentolamine
		Epinephrine (adrenaline)	Doxazosin
		Norepinephrine (noradrenaline)	Prazosin
	α_2-Adrenoceptor	Clonidine	Phentolamine
		Brimonidine	
	β_1-Adrenoceptor	Epinephrine (adrenaline)	Propanolol
		Isoprenaline	Atenolol
		Dobutamine	Bisoprolol
	β_2-Adrenoceptor	Salbutamol, terbutaline	Propranolol
			Timolol
	$5\text{-}HT_1$	Sumatriptan	Methysergide
	$5\text{-}HT_3$	—	Ondansetron
	Dopamine D_2	Bromocriptine	Domperidone
		Lysuride	Metoclopramide
		Pergolide	Chlorpromazine
	Histamine H_1	—	Chlorpheniramine
	Histamine H_2	—	Cimetidine, ranitidine
	Mineralocorticoid	Fludrocortisone	Spironolactone
	Vasopressin	Glypressin	—
	Somatostatin	Octreotide	—
	Angiotensin II	—	Losartan
	Platelet glycoprotein IIb/IIIa	—	Abciximab
	Cysteinyl leukotriene	—	Montelukast, zafirlukast
Enzyme	*Target*	*Inhibitor*	
	Cholinesterase	Neostigmine	
		Pyridostigmine	
		Edrophonium	
		Dorepeid (CE: AQ)	
	Cyclo-oxygenase (COX)	Aspirin, NSAIDs	
	COX-2	Rofecoxib, celecoxib	
	Xanthine oxidase	Allopurinol	
	ACE	Captopril, enalpril, lisinopril	
	HMG-CoA reducatse	Simvastatin, pravastatin	
	MAO-A	Pargyline, isocarboxazid, moclobemide	
	MAO-B	Selegeline	
Carriers	Uptake 1	Tricyclics, cocaine	
	Weak acids	Probenecid	
	$Na^+/K^+/Cl^-$ co-transporter	Furosemide (frusemide), bumetanide	
	Na^+/K^+-ATPase	Digoxin	
	H^+-ATPase	Omeprazole	

ACE, angiotensin-converting enzyme; ACh, acetylcholine; HMG, hydroxymethylglutaryl; HT, hydroxytyptamine; MAO, monoamine oxidase; NMJ, neuromuscular junction; NSAIDs, non-steroidal anti-inflammatory drugs.

Not all drugs target proteins. Examples of those that do not include the following:
- general anaesthetics act by altering the properties of the lipid membrane of neurons
- oxygen (an important and widely prescribed drug) receives electrons transported along the mitochondrial respiratory chain as part of cellular respiration
- lactulose (which is not absorbed) and mannitol (which is absorbed) act by altering the osmotic balance in the bowel lumen and vascular compartment, respectively
- antacids neutralize gastric contents
- cholestyramine, a bile-acid-binding resin, lowers cholesterol by inhibiting its enterohepatic recirculation.

Knowing the nature of the drug target and its role in normal physiology allows some predictions to be made about the amount of drug required to exert an effect and how quickly the effect will occur. Drugs that target membrane surface receptors for hormones or neurotransmitters have a rapid action, particularly if the drug is delivered by the intravenous route and targets a surface receptor that is coupled to a rapidly acting signal transduction cascade or an ion channel. For other drugs, although the interaction of the drug with its target may be rapid, the onset of the therapeutic effect can be delayed because the kinetics of the system that is affected are slow.

Example 9: Rapid treatment of a rapid pulse

Case history
A fit 30-year-old woman with a history of episodic self-terminating palpitations attends the A&E department with a further, more prolonged episode. She is haemodynamically stable and her ECG reveals a regular, narrow, complex tachycardia with a rate of 180/min. Carotid sinus massage is ineffective. (See *Cardiology*, Sections 1.1, 1.2 and 2.2.2.)

Clinical approach
The probable diagnosis here is of an atrioventricular re-entrant or atrioventricular nodal re-entrant tachycardia (AVRT or AVNRT), the substrate being a re-entrant circuit involving the atrioventricular (AV) node. These dysrhythmias can therefore be terminated by producing transient AV nodal blockade of even a few seconds' duration. Vagotonic manoeuvres (e.g. carotid sinus massage) are usually tried first but, if ineffective, the drug of choice is adenosine, which binds G-protein-coupled adenosine receptors on the surface of conducting cells in the AV node. This action results in the rapid opening of membrane K^+ channels, hyperpolarization and conduction block. When given by fast intravenous injection, the onset of effect is rapid, occurring within seconds. Furthermore, the effects of adenosine are extremely short-lived because the drug is rapidly removed from the circulation by carrier-mediated uptake and metabolism in endothelial cells. Rapid uptake and inactivation do not compromise the effect of the drug and are, in fact, advantageous because they minimize side effects. It does mean, however, that the drug must be administered by fast intravenous bolus.

Example 10: Thyrotoxicosis: how fast will it get better?

Case history
A 61-year-old woman with a 6-month history of weight loss, palpitations, tremor and heat intolerance is diagnosed as having primary thyrotoxicosis caused by Graves' disease. She is concerned about whether her treatment will result in the prompt resolution of symptoms. (See *Endocrinology*, Sections 1.13 and 2.3.2.)

Example 10: Thyrotoxicosis: how fast will it get better? (*continued*)

Clinical approach
The aims of treatment are to relieve symptoms and to render the patient euthyroid. Thionamides (e.g. carbimazole and propylthiouracil) inhibit the formation of thyroid hormones by interfering with the incorporation of iodine into the tyrosyl residues of thyroglobulin. This is achieved by inhibition of the peroxidase enzyme, which catalyses this reaction. Synthesis of new hormone is inhibited, but the full therapeutic effect may not be seen until the stores of preformed hormone have been depleted, which can take 6–8 weeks. During this time, the symptoms of tremor and palpitations can be treated by a non-selective β blocker such as propranolol. In the long term, the definitive treatment of this woman's condition might be with radioiodine.

Grahame-Smith DG, Aronson JK. *Oxford Textbook of Clinical Pharmacology and Drug Therapy*, 2nd edn. Oxford: Oxford University Press, 1992.

3.2 Selectivity is the key to the therapeutic utility of an agent

For a drug to be clinically useful, it should be capable of modifying a particular function in a particular cell or tissue without altering related or unrelated functions elsewhere in the body. In the best case, the action of a drug would be restricted solely to the target organ or tissue. Rather inconveniently, many of the common targets for drugs, such as membrane receptors or ion channels, are widely distributed, often in diverse organs or tissues (Fig. 13). For this reason, the therapeutic goal of absolute selectivity is, in practice, difficult to attain.

Selectivity of action from localized delivery of a drug

On occasion, the aim of selectivity can be achieved by delivery of the drug locally to its desired site of action. This is feasible for drugs that act on the skin, eye, airways, and upper and lower gastrointestinal tract. However, if significant absorption occurs from the site of local delivery, systemic side effects may still result.

Example 11: A systemic effect of local treatment

Case history
A 74-year-old woman who smokes is found by her optician to have an intraocular pressure of 28 mmHg in both eyes, an arcuate visual field defect, and disc cupping compatible with a diagnosis of primary open-angle glaucoma. After ophthalmological referral, she is prescribed timolol eye drops. At the 6-week follow-up the intraocular pressure in both eyes has fallen to 19 mmHg, but she complains of tiredness, low mood and difficulty climbing stairs. Respiratory examination reveals bilateral polyphonic wheezes and her peak expiratory flow rate is 150 L/min.

Clinical approach
This patient is likely to be manifesting side effects from timolol, a non-selective β blocker that may be absorbed from the ocular surface and block β-receptors in the lungs and brain (Figs 13 and 14). β₂-Adrenoceptor blockade in the small airways may unmask an undiagnosed asthmatic component to chronic obstructive airway disease in a smoker, and many studies have documented worsening of pulmonary function in elderly patients treated with timolol eye drops, although the incidence of frank respiratory symptoms is low. Timolol is also lipid soluble and can therefore cross the blood–brain barrier, where symptoms arising from β blockade include tiredness, depression, poor sleep and nightmares. Fortunately, alternative treatments are available for the treatment of primary open-angle glaucoma and include brimonidine (an α₂-adrenoceptor agonist), dorzolamide (a carbonic anhydrase inhibitor), latanoprost (a prostaglandin analogue) and pilocarpine (a muscarinic cholinoceptor agonist).

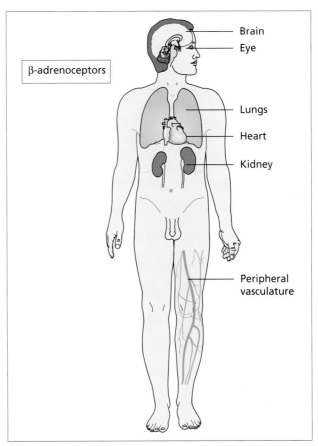

Fig. 13 Some drug targets are distributed widely. β-Adrenoceptors can be found in the brain, eye, lungs, heart, kidney and blood vessels.

Corticosteroids are commonly administered locally to limit systemic side effects. Sites of delivery include the ocular surface (for allergic and inflammatory eye disease), the airways (for asthma), the skin (for eczema) and the rectum and colon (for ulcerative colitis and Crohn's disease). However, suppression of adrenocortical function and effects on bone mineral metabolism may still be observed, particularly if high dosages are used.

Pharmacological selectivity

Selectivity of action is most commonly achieved by using drugs with a particular affinity for receptor, channel or enzyme subtypes, the expression of which is restricted to the cells or tissue of interest. In the best case, the concentration of drug required to modify the target receptor subtype may be many orders of magnitude lower than that at which related receptor subtypes are bound. However, complete selectivity is rarely achieved and many of the adverse effects of drugs result from their interaction with related receptors, enzymes or ion channels located at distant sites.

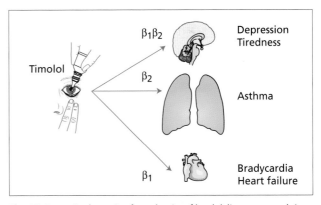

Fig. 14 Systemic absorption from the site of local delivery can result in side effects.

Example 12: Unwanted dizziness

Case history
A 78-year-old man with hesitancy, poor urinary stream and nocturia is diagnosed as having bladder outflow tract obstruction from benign prostatic hyperplasia. He is prescribed doxazosin with good relief of his urinary symptoms, but he complains of dizziness on standing, particularly when getting out of bed in the morning. (See *Medicine for the elderly*, Section 1.1.)

Example 12: Unwanted dizziness (*continued*)

Clinical approach
In benign prostatic hyperplasia, urinary outflow obstruction is partly structural and partly functional. The functional component results from tonic α_1-adrenoceptor-mediated contraction of smooth muscle in the bladder neck, prostatic capsule and prostatic urethra. α_1-Adrenoceptor antagonists (such as prazosin, doxazosin and terazosin) improve symptoms in this disorder by causing relaxation of smooth muscle at these sites. The major side effect of this group of drugs is postural hypotension caused by blockade of α_1-adrenoceptors in the smooth muscle of small arteries, which results in a reduction in peripheral resistance and hence a fall in blood pressure (Fig. 15). Guidance about rising slowly from a lying position or when getting out of a chair may be all that is required. Finasteride (a 5α-reductase inhibitor that prevents the conversion of testosterone to dihydrotestosterone and reduces prostatic volume) could be used as an alternative to doxazosin. Its therapeutic effects are seen after several months of therapy.

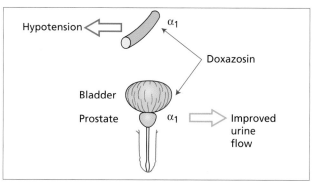

Fig. 15 Binding of a drug to its target results in the therapeutic response, but binding to related proteins elsewhere can lead to side effects.

Traditionally, receptor subtypes were classified in functional terms on the basis of similarities and differences in response to agonists and antagonists (see below). More recently, with the advent of recombinant DNA technology, receptors have come to be redefined in structural terms on the basis of their DNA and amino acid sequences. Related receptors (receptor families) are sometimes the products of distinct but structurally similar genes or, occasionally, are encoded by the same gene with structural differences introduced at the level of mRNA processing.

Example 13: A patient who had not read the latest papers

Case history
A 58-year-old man with stable New York Heart Association (NYHA) grade III heart failure from dilated cardiomyopathy, treated with furosemide (frusemide) and ramipril, is started on a low dose of bisoprolol in the light of recent studies that have demonstrated mortality reductions with low-dose β blockade in patients with mild to moderate heart failure. One week after the start of treatment, he complains of breathlessness and a chest radiograph shows upper lobe blood diversion and Kerley B lines. (See *Cardiology*, Section 1.6.)

Clinical approach
Patients with heart failure exhibit compensatory activation of the sympathetic nervous system, which helps maintain cardiac output in the face of impaired myocardial performance. In the long term, this heightened sympathetic drive may have deleterious effects on cardiac myocytes and may promote dysrhythmias. The mechanism by which β blockers reduce mortality in patients with heart failure is unknown, but may be related to an antiarrhythmic effect mediated by blockade of β$_1$-adrenoceptors on myocardial cells and in conducting tissue. β Blockers should be started at low dose in patients with heart failure, because their negative inotropic effect may result in a rapid reduction in cardiac output, worsening heart failure and even pulmonary oedema.

Example 13: A patient who had not read the latest papers (*continued*)

Any dosage increase should be made slowly and conducted under specialist supervision. If there is a deterioration in the symptoms or signs of heart failure, the dose of β blocker should be reduced and the dose of diuretic and angiotensin-converting enzyme (ACE) inhibitor increased (if possible). A subsequent increase in the dose of β blocker (to the maintenance dosage used in recent trials) may then be possible.

 When using β blockers in patients with heart failure, be aware of the narrow therapeutic window.
- Ensure that the condition is stable and that the patient has heart failure in NYHA grade II or III
- Use bisoprolol, metoprolol or carvedilol (currently the only β blocker licensed for this indication in the UK) because these are the agents that have been evaluated in clinical trials
- Start at a low dose and titrate the dose upwards with care ('START LOW, GO SLOW'); the daily dosing schedule for carvedilol is: 3.125 mg initially, increasing to 6.25 mg after 1 week, 12.5 mg after 3 weeks, 25 mg after 5 weeks and 50 mg after 7 weeks
- Ensure frequent follow-up and active monitoring for clinical deterioration.

CIBIS II Investigators and Committee. *Lancet* 1999; 353: 9–13.
Packer M *et al. N Engl J Med* 1996; 334: 1349–55.
Waagstein F *et al. Lancet* 1993; 342: 1442–6.

3.3 Basic aspects of a drug's interaction with its target

Agonists and the dose–response curve

Many of the principles of drug action were developed around the interaction of drug molecules with membrane receptors. The term 'agonist' is given to a drug that binds to a receptor to produce the same biological response as the receptor's natural ligand. In most cases, the binding of a drug to its receptor is a reversible process and the degree of receptor activation, which is related to the number of receptors that are bound by a drug at any one time, is proportional to the concentration of drug in the vicinity of the receptor. A graph that depicts the relationship between the logarithm of the concentration of an agonist drug and the proportion of the maximal biological effect produced is called a log concentration–response curve and is sigmoid in shape. As the concentration of drug is related to the dose administered, the terms 'concentration–response curve' and 'dose–response curve' are sometimes used interchangeably (Fig. 16).

For some drugs, the dose administered provides a local concentration close to that required for the maximal therapeutic response (Fig. 16). For this reason, increasing the dose of drug confers no additional therapeutic benefit and may increase the likelihood of side effects, the incidence of which may be more closely dependent on dose (Fig. 17).

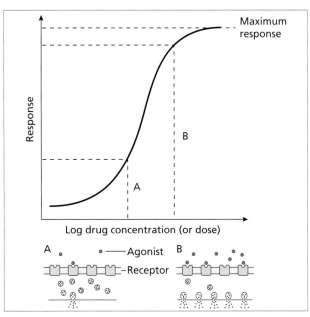

Fig. 16 Relationship between drug dose and response. Increasing the concentration of drug (A–B) results in an enhanced response.

Example 14: A man who decides to take double the dose

Case history
A 65-year-old man with uncomplicated essential hypertension is prescribed bendrofluazide 2.5 mg daily by his GP, and elects to purchase an automated home blood pressure-recording device. After several BP recordings of around 165/105, he decides to double the dose of bendrofluazide. On review in the surgery 4 weeks later, his BP is 168/108 and his serum K^+ 2.2 mmol/L. (See *Cardiology*, Section 1.15.)

Clinical approach
In this patient, the increase in dose of bendrofluazide from 2.5 mg to 5 mg fails to produce a reduction in BP but, instead, results in hypokalaemia. Other metabolic side effects of bendrofluazide (e.g. hyperglycaemia, hyperuricaemia and elevations in serum lipids) are also more common with higher doses. For patients whose BP remains poorly controlled with low-dose bendrofluazide, introduction of a second antihypertensive agent (e.g. a β blocker or ACE inhibitor), the actions of which are synergistic with those of the thiazide diuretic, will usually result in adequate BP control with fewer side effects.

Potency, efficacy and partial agonists

A potent agonist drug is one that is capable of producing the maximal response from a tissue at a low concentration. Ultimately, the maximum possible biological response that can be elicited from a tissue is determined not by the potency of the drug but by the capacity of the tissue to respond. For instance, once the receptors that activate the secretion of a neurotransmitter are maximally

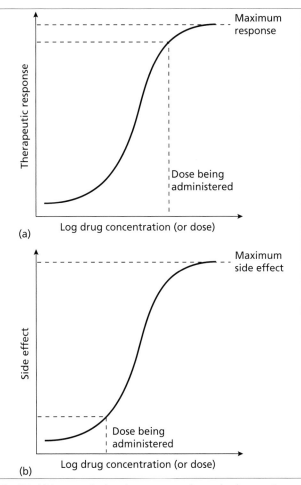

Fig. 17 (a) Increases in drug dose may not enhance the therapeutic response, if the dose being administered already lies close to the top of the dose–response curve. (b) Instead, it may lead to more side effects.

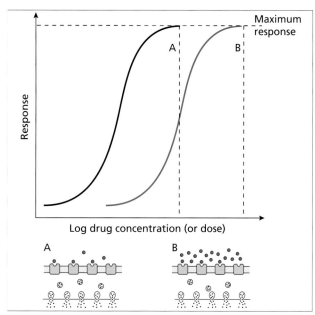

Fig. 18 A drug of lower potency (B) elicits the same maximum response as a drug of high potency (A), provided that a higher dose is used.

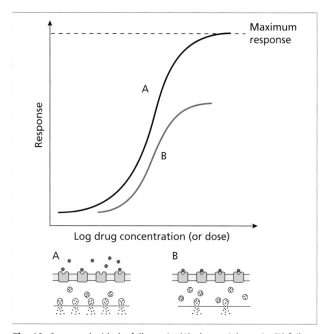

Fig. 19 Compared with the full agonist (A), the partial agonist (B) fails to elicit the maximum response despite full receptor occupancy.

bound by their activating ligand, the maximum amount of neurotransmitter released will be determined by the level of the intracellular stores. For this reason, a drug of low potency is capable of producing the same maximum response as a highly potent drug, provided that it is administered at a higher dose (Fig. 18).

In clinical practice, the potency of the drug is less important than its efficacy, which refers to the maximum response that a drug elicits when all its target receptors are occupied. Some agonist drugs fail to elicit a maximal response despite maximum receptor occupancy (Fig. 19).

Such drugs are called partial agonists. In the presence of a full agonist, a partial agonist can have antagonist effects because it competes with the full agonist for occupation of a receptor, but fails to elicit the same degree of response.

Example 15: Addition of a new drug may have a subtractive effect

Case history
A 55-year-old man is receiving morphine subcutaneously through a continuous infusion device for postoperative analgesia after a sigmoid colectomy. Pain control is suboptimal and the patient requests sublingual buprenorphine, which he has used in the past to good effect. (See *Pain relief and palliative care*, Sections 1.1 and 2.1.)

Clinical approach
Both morphine and buprenorphine are opiate analgesics that target the μ-opioid receptor in the central nervous system (CNS). Morphine is a full agonist at this receptor, but buprenorphine is a partial agonist. Although an effective analgesic on its own, buprenorphine would be expected to antagonize the action of morphine and may, in this instance, worsen the pain control. The strategy here should be to define more precisely the nature of the pain, to exclude immediately remediable causes such as a poorly sited urinary catheter and, if necessary, to increase the morphine dose.

Antagonists

Some drugs achieve their effect by binding and occupying a receptor without activating it. In so doing they inhibit the binding of the natural ligand to the receptor and attenuate the normal biological function. Many drugs of this type are in clinical use (see Table 13), most being reversible competitive antagonists, meaning that their binding to the target receptor is reversible and that they compete with the natural ligand for receptor occupancy. Their effect is to increase the concentration of natural ligand required to produce a given response, so the effect of the antagonist can be overcome by increases in the concentration of the natural ligand (Fig. 20). Another feature of such drugs is that their effect is dependent on the degree of activation of the pathway, of which the receptor is part—the more active the pathway, the greater the biological effect of the antagonist (Fig. 20).

Competitive antagonists are also used as antidotes to counteract the action of a second drug, including drugs that have been taken as part of a deliberate overdose. Examples include naloxone (a μ-opiate receptor antagonist used in the diagnosis and treatment of heroin overdose) and flumazenil (a γ-aminobutyric acid or GABA receptor antagonist used in the diagnosis and treatment of benzodiazepine overdose).

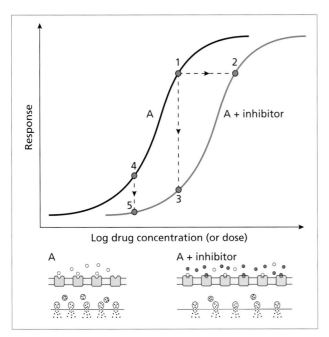

Fig. 20 In the presence of a competitive inhibitor, the concentration–response curve for the endogenous ligand A is shifted to the right. With a higher concentration of ligand A (point 1 to point 2), the effect of the inhibitor can be overcome and the same response can be attained. When a system is highly active (point 1 vs point 4), the effect of an inhibitor is greater (compare the large change in response from point 1 to point 3 with the change from point 4 to point 5).

Example 16: Too much benzodiazepine

Case history
A 79-year-old woman, recently widowed, is brought to the A&E department as an emergency. She is unconscious with a Glasgow Coma Score of 8/15, but is breathing spontaneously with a Guedel airway *in situ* and a respiratory rate of 16/min. Her pulse rate is 80/min and BP 144/86 mmHg. There is no evidence of meningeal irritation and there are no focal neurological signs or signs of head injury. An empty bottle of temazepam tablets was found in her purse. Flumazenil 1 mg intravenously produces a prompt, complete but short-lived reversal of unconsciousness. (See *Emergency medicine*, Sections 1.26 and 2.1.)

Clinical approach
This woman exhibits the features of a major benzodiazepine overdose. The CNS depressant effects of this drug can be reversed by flumazenil, which can be used to make the diagnosis of benzodiazepine overdose and exclude other toxic/metabolic causes of coma. The effects of flumazenil are short-lived because its half-life (1 h) is much shorter than that of temazepam (about 11 h). Sedation may return, and appropriate measures to support breathing and circulation need to be taken while the benzodiazepine is metabolized.

Flumazenil should be used cautiously in combined overdose of benzodiazepines and tricyclic antidepressants. Under these circumstances, the benzodiazepine may be helping to suppress seizure activity resulting from tricyclic overdose, and flumazenil can precipitate seizure.

Opioid overdose and naloxone

The half-life of the opioid antagonist naloxone is much shorter than that of most of the opiates encountered in overdose. Transient reversal of respiratory depression, sedation and coma by a bolus dose of naloxone may provide the patient and physician with a false sense of security, because respiratory depression may return as the naloxone is metabolized. Patients should be advised to remain under close observation and respiratory support provided if required. A continuous infusion of naloxone may be needed.

Physiological antagonism

Some agents interfere with the action of a natural ligand or another drug, not by blocking its receptor but by increasing the activity of a separate system or pathway that has an opposing action. Such a process is termed 'physiological antagonism'.

The phenomenon of physiological antagonism may be used to good effect in patients who develop hypoglycaemia after overdose with insulin. This can be treated by 50 mL of 50% dextrose intravenously or—if venous access is difficult—by 1 mg glucagon by intramuscular injection. Glucagon causes glycogenolysis and mobilization of hepatic glucose stores which reverse the hypoglycaemia—an example of physiological antagonism.

Glucagon also finds use as a physiological antagonist in the management of severe β-blocker overdose. The manifestations of such an overdose include bronchospasm (which can be treated by nebulized salbutamol), bradycardia (which is treated by temporary pacing or atropine, in another example of physiological antagonism) and hypotension caused by the direct negative inotropic effects of β blockers. In this situation glucagon, given by intravenous infusion, binds its receptors on the myocardium and increases intracellular concentrations of cAMP (cyclic adenosine 3′:5′-monophosphate), thus opposing the negative inotropic effects of β blockade.

Inhibitors and blockers

Membrane receptors are not the only targets for drugs that interfere with a natural function. Drugs that inhibit the function of enzymes are referred to as inhibitors and drugs that inhibit the function of ion channels as blockers. Enzyme inhibition and channel blockade can also be reversible or irreversible.

Those drugs that inhibit enzymes irreversibly can have biological effects, the duration of which persists long after withdrawal. Examples include aspirin (whose antiplatelet effect is mediated by irreversible inhibition of cyclo-oxygenase) and the traditional irreversible monoamine oxidase (MAO) inhibitors, which are used as antidepressants. These drugs may need to be stopped before surgery (as aspirin can potentiate blood loss, and MAO inhibitors have adverse interactions with certain anaesthetic agents); if so, aspirin should be withdrawn about 10 days preoperatively and MAO inhibitors 2–3 weeks before surgery. A reversible inhibitor of MAO-A (a RIMA, e.g. moclobemide) can be used as an alternative antidepressant during this time.

Tolerance: why drug effects sometimes wane

The effect of a drug sometimes lessens with continued use. Tachyphylaxis, desensitization or tolerance are terms used, sometimes interchangeably, to describe this phenomenon. The mechanisms underlying tolerance are varied and may be pharmacokinetic (the result of enhanced drug metabolism) or pharmacodynamic (the result of changes in receptor numbers or the sensitivity of postreceptor signalling mechanisms). Sometimes tolerance arises from an adaptive response of a tissue caused by the upregulation of a counter-regulatory system.

Patients receiving organic nitrates for angina develop tolerance to their effects with dose regimens that sustain plasma or tissue nitrate concentrations for more than a 24-h period. The mechanisms underlying nitrate tolerance are unknown, but it has been suggested that depletion of tissue sulphydryl or thiol groups (which are necessary for the effects of nitrates), increased generation of antioxidants or reflex activation of the renin–angiotensin system may all play a part. The only measure shown to be effective in preventing nitrate tolerance is the use of a dosing schedule that gives a nitrate-free interval during some part of the day.

Ross EM. Pharmacodynamics: mechanisms of drug action and the relationship between drug concentration and effect. In: Hardman JG, Limbird LE, eds. *Goodman and Gilman's Pharmacological Basis of Therapeutics*, 9th edn. New York: McGraw-Hill, 1996: 29–41.

3.4 Heterogeneity of drug responses, pharmacogenetics and pharmacogenomics

One drug does not fit all.
(Andrew Marshall, *Nature Biotechnology*, October 1998)

Most clinicians are aware that certain patients respond better to some drugs than others. This is particularly true for disorders such as hypertension, where the underlying pathophysiology is unknown and different classes of drug are often tried sequentially until an adequate therapeutic response is achieved. Just as common variation in the sequence of certain key genes (polymorphisms) can influence the way that different individuals metabolize drugs (see Table 8), so it is possible that polymorphisms in other genes might influence pharmacodynamic responses through effects on the expression or activity of receptors, ion channels or enzymes.

Pharmacogenetics

Pharmacogenetics is the study of genetically determined variations in drug metabolism. It is clinically important because pharmacogenetic variation underlies certain adverse drug reactions, and results in clinically important variations in response to commonly prescribed drugs and hence unexpected toxicity or therapeutic failure.

Pharmacogenomics

'Pharmacogenomics' is the term given to an emerging discipline that aims to identify genetic determinants of pharmacodynamic responses and to use this information to guide therapy and limit side effects. It is still in its infancy and there are currently few examples of its utility.

An illustration of the potential importance of pharmacogenomics is provided by individuals with a common mutation in the gene for factor V (factor V Leiden), who are resistant to the fibrinolytic actions of activated protein C and at high risk of venous thromboembolic disease. In women with this mutation who are exposed to the third-generation combined oral contraceptive pill, which contains progestogens that reduce activated protein C activity, there is an interaction between these two risk factors that causes a substantial magnification of the thromboembolic risk.

4   Adverse drug reactions

4.1 Introduction

Adverse drug reactions and interactions are common. At least 5% of all acute medical admissions to hospital are caused by adverse effects of drugs (not including deliberate self-harm), and up to 20% of all hospital inpatients are subject to significant drug-related illness; in half of them, this will prolong their period of stay in hospital. In the USA, it has been calculated that one in seven of all hospital beds are taken up for the treatment of adverse reactions resulting from drugs. The morbidity, mortality and cost of drug-related disease are therefore considerable.

There is an increasing range of therapeutically valuable drugs available in modern clinical practice, and the potential for adverse reactions and interactions is almost unlimited. Every prescriber must be aware of the potential for drug-induced disease and must have a good understanding of the more common mechanisms that underlie adverse drug reactions. Only by understanding the mechanisms involved can the incidence of adverse reactions be minimized, and when they do occur early action taken to avert more serious consequences. All decisions about prescribing involve undertaking a risk–benefit analysis. Always consider the damage that your intervention might cause for the individual patient concerned and weigh this against the likely benefit (Fig. 21).

If in doubt about a drug with which you are not absolutely familiar, LOOK IT UP.

Medicine is a collection of uncertain prescriptions which kill the poor, and succeed sometimes with the rich; and the results of which, collectively taken, are more fatal than useful to mankind. Speak to me no more about these fine things; I am not a man for drugs. (Napoleon Bonaparte [1769–1821])

Example 17: Should you risk harm while trying to do good?

Case history
An 87-year-old woman is admitted after a series of falls which are thought to be related to her poor visual acuity and advanced osteoarthritis. She is found to have mild heart failure with mitral regurgitation and atrial fibrillation, and the question is raised of whether she should receive anticoagulation with warfarin to protect against emboli. What are the likely risks and benefits of this and how would you make your decision? (See *Neurology*, Sections 2.8.1 and 2.8.2.)

Clinical approach
The combination of atrial fibrillation, heart failure and mitral regurgitation places this woman at high risk of stroke and there is good evidence that adjusted-dose warfarin provides the best risk reduction in this circumstance. However, in view of her impaired visual acuity and propensity to falls, what do you think the risks are for this particular patient and how do they match up against any theoretical benefit? In this circumstance, the risks probably outweigh the benefits.

Briggs GG, Freeman RK, Yaffe SJ. *Drugs in Pregnancy and Lactation*, 5th edn. Baltimore: Williams & Williams, 1998.

Davies DM, Ferner RE, Glanville H de, eds. *Davies's Textbook of Adverse Drug Reactions*, 5th edn. London: Chapman & Hall, 1998.

Dukes MNG, Aronson JK. *Meyler's Side Effects of Drugs*, 14th edn. Amsterdam: Elsevier, 2000.

Hallas J, Gram LF, Grodum E *et al.* Drug related admissions to medical wards: a population based survey. *Br J Clin Pharmacol* 1992; 33: 61–8.

Stroke Prevention in Atrial Fibrillation Investigators. Adjusted dose warfarin vs. low intensity, fixed dose warfarin plus aspirin for high-risk patients with atrial fibrillation: Stroke Prevention in Atrial Fibrillation III randomized clinical trial. *Lancet* 1996; 348: 633–8.

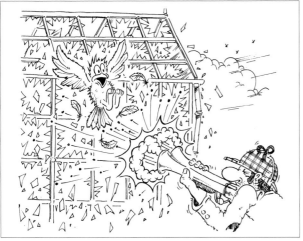

Fig. 21 Always make a risk–benefit assessment before you prescribe.

4.2 Definition and classification of adverse drug reactions

An adverse drug reaction is any unwanted effect of a drug that arises at doses normally used in the treatment, diagnosis or prevention of disease (Table 14). This definition therefore excludes drug overdoses arising from the administration (intentionally or otherwise) of doses greater than those normally used therapeutically.

Table 14 The classification of adverse drug reactions.

Dose-related effects (type A reactions)
Non-dose-related effects (type B reactions)
Long-term effects
Delayed effects

Certain factors may predispose to adverse drug reactions:
- Age: adverse reactions are more common at the extremes of age
- Sex: women are at greater risk
- Race: pharmacogenetic variations form the basis for many adverse reactions
- History of atopy or allergic disorders
- History of a previous adverse drug reaction
- Renal impairment
- Hepatic impairment
- Heart failure
- Nutritional status: the overweight and undernourished are at greater risk
- Multiple drug therapy.

> The greater number of simples that go unto anie compound medicine, the greater the confusion is found therein, because the qualities and operations of verie few of the particular are thoroughlie knowne. (William Harrison [1534–1593])

4.3 Dose-related adverse drug reactions

These arise from an exaggeration of the predictable effects of a drug and are most commonly seen with drugs that have a narrow therapeutic range. They occur largely because of pharmacokinetic or pharmacodynamic variability from the norm (see Fig. 8).

> Poisons and medicine are oftentimes the same substance given with different intents.
> (Peter Mere Latham [1789–1875])

Example 18: A cause of confusion

Case history
A 79-year-old woman with type 2 (non-insulin-dependent) diabetes taking glibenclamide 10 mg a day is failing to cope at home and has fallen several times. Initially this was attributed to a urinary infection, treated by her GP with trimethoprim, but now she has become acutely confused. (See *Medicine for the elderly*, Sections 1.1 and 1.2.)

Clinical approach
The cause of this woman's falls and recent confusion was thought to be hypoglycaemia, after her blood glucose on admission to hospital was found to be 2.1 mmol/L. Why had her normally good glycaemic control on a stable dose of glibenclamide recently become problematic?

Glibenclamide undergoes hepatic metabolism and its active metabolites are renally excreted. Hence, in patients with renal impairment, the effect of glibenclamide is exaggerated. In this case the patient had developed a moderate degree of renal impairment with a creatinine of 195 µmol/L and the steady accumulation of her sulphonylurea led to symptomatic hypoglycaemia. In addition to this, there is an interaction between trimethoprim and glibenclamide which can result in an enhanced hypoglycaemic effect. Avoid long-acting drugs that can accumulate in renal failure, such as chlorpropramide and glibenclamide, but consider drugs with a short half-life and that undergo a significant degree of hepatic elimination, e.g. glipizide.

Examples of dose-related adverse drug reactions

Excess of the intended therapeutic action:
- Hypoglycaemia caused by sulphonylureas
- Hypotension caused by vasodilator drugs
- Dehydration caused by diuretics
- Symptomatic bradycardia caused by β blockers
- Haemorrhage caused by anticoagulants
- Hypothyroidism caused by antithyroid drugs.
Pharmacological actions unrelated to the desired therapeutic effect:
- Gout caused by thiazide diuretics
- Anticholinergic effects of tricyclic antidepressants
- Ototoxicity of aminoglycosides
- Gastrointestinal bleeding caused by non-steroidal anti-inflammatory drugs
- Nephrotoxicity of cyclosporin.

Pharmacogenetic variation as a cause of dose-related adverse drug reactions

Metabolism can terminate the effect of a drug, generate active metabolites that are therapeutically important or generate metabolites that contribute to adverse effects. In general the enzymes that are involved in drug metabolism are typified by the following:
- broad substrate specificity
- affinity for endogenous and exogenous substrates
- multiple forms (isoenzymes)
- species differences.

The major site of drug metabolism is in the liver and some metabolic pathways are subject to genetic polymorphism (see Table 8). Three examples are discussed below.

Cytochrome P450 2D6

A number of clinically important drugs are oxidized principally by one isoenzyme of cytochrome P450: CYP 2D6 (see Table 8), a route of metabolism also known as the sparteine/debrisoquine oxidative pathway. The activity of CYP 2D6 is largely genetically determined, and the general European population segregates into two phenotypes: extensive metabolizers (90–95%) and poor metabolizers (5–10%). Poor metabolizers are homozygous for an autosomal recessive allele and extensive metabolizers are homozygous dominants or heterozygous. Poor metabolizers have no CYP 2D6 activity.

The clinical relevance of the CYP 2D6 polymorphism is most apparent for drugs that have a relatively low therapeutic : toxic ratio. If metoprolol is given in standard doses to a poor metabolizer, it may cause excessive β blockade; in the case of the tricyclic antidepressants, there is a greater risk of adverse effects in poor metabolizers as a result of the anticholinergic properties of these drugs. Codeine is a prodrug that is metabolized to morphine by CYP 2D6; poor metabolizers cannot perform this conversion and may therefore not achieve adequate analgesia if treated with codeine.

Drug acetylation

In the early 1950s, it was noticed that there was a large variation in the metabolism of the antituberculous drug isoniazid, and distribution histograms of the percentage of isoniazid excreted unchanged in the urine showed a bimodal distribution. Isoniazid is metabolized in the liver by a process of acetylation and this bimodal distribution suggested that individuals are either fast or slow acetylators. Acetylator status is inherited in a simple mendelian manner, slow acetylators being autosomal recessive homozygotes and fast acetylators heterozygotes or autosomal dominant homozygotes. There are marked differences in the relative proportions of slow and fast acetylators in different races.

Table 15 Dose-related adverse drug reactions arising from slow acetylator status.

Drug	Drug class	Adverse reaction
Isoniazid	Antibacterial	Peripheral neuropathy
Procainamide	Antiarrythmic	Lupus-like syndrome
Hydralazine	Vasodilator	Lupus-like syndrome
Sulphasalazine	Sulphonamide	Haemolysis
Dapsone	Sulphonamide	Haemolysis
Phenelzine	MAO inhibitor	MAO inhibitor toxicity

MAO, monoamine oxidase.

Acetylator status is not only relevant to isoniazid; other drugs of clinical significance are inactivated by the same enzymatic process (Table 15).

The significance of acetylator status for adverse drug reactions is that slow acetylators will achieve a higher plasma concentration of drug for a given dose than fast acetylators. Although this may result in a greater therapeutic effect (as in the antihypertensive effect of hydralazine), it also gives rise to adverse effects at dosages normally used in the treatment of disease. By contrast to slow acetylators, there is a suggestion that fast acetylators may be more at risk of isoniazid-induced hepatitis because the acetylated metabolite, acetylhydrazine, is further metabolized to a potent alkylating agent, which can covalently bind to liver cells.

Thiopurine methyltransferase

Example 19: 'Over-immunosuppression'

Case history
A 43-year-old man undergoes renal transplantation for end-stage renal disease and is immunosuppressed with appropriate doses of ciclosporin, azathioprine and prednisolone. After transplantation he develops a rapidly progressive pancytopenia. (See *Immunology and immunosuppression*, Section 8 and *Nephrology*, Section 2.2.3.)

Clinical approach
Azathioprine is converted to the active cytotoxic metabolite 6-mercaptopurine. Pancytopenia caused by marrow toxicity is a well-recognized complication of therapy with azathioprine and other thiopurines. The rapid progression of severe pancytopenia at appropriate therapeutic doses of azathioprine should alert you to the possibilities of a drug interaction, or a pharmacogenetic idiosyncrasy resulting in increased exposure to the cytotoxic metabolite of azathioprine. A close examination of the drug chart will reveal any co-prescribed medications that might be implicated. The dose of azathioprine should be carefully checked.

Azathioprine is a synthetic nucleotide used extensively in organ transplantation and autoimmune disease. The metabolism of azathioprine and related thiopurines (6-mercaptopurine and 6-thioguanine) is the result of the action of two enzymes—xanthine oxidase and thiopurine methyltransferase (TPMT) (Fig. 22). A deficiency in the activity of either enzyme could result in the accumulation of toxic metabolites that produce profound marrow suppression. Allopurinol is known to inhibit xanthine oxidase, and significant reductions in the dose of azathioprine are required when the two drugs are co-prescribed. Low activity of TPMT is inherited as a rare autosomal recessive trait (1 in 300 Caucasians; 11% prevalence of the heterozygous state), and the administration of appropriate therapeutic doses of azathioprine to such individuals results in severe marrow toxicity. This patient was found to be a low TPMT metabolizer by polymerase chain reaction (PCR)-based analysis; azathioprine was withdrawn and his marrow gradually recovered.

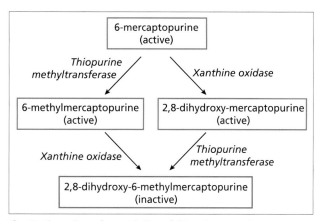

Fig. 22 The pathway for metabolism of thiopurine cytotoxic agents.

Is it worth screening for drug metabolizer status?

The clinical scenario presented in example 19 could have been prevented by pre-screening for autosomal recessive TPMT deficiency. However, given the close monitoring of patients after commencement of azathioprine therapy, the rarity of the condition and high cost of screening, this approach is not employed at present.

What about the future?

Many in academia and industry think that genetic profiling of patients for all pharmacogenetic variables will become a reality within 20 years. If so, general practitioners and hospital practitioners will need to have access to this information for all patients and be expected to use it to aid their prescribing.

Dose-related drug–disease interaction

Example 20: More trouble with the foxglove

Case history
A 74-year-old woman with a long-standing atrial fibrillation controlled with digoxin 250 µg/day develops mild heart failure; her GP gives her furosemide (frusemide) at a dose of 40 mg/day. Six weeks later she complains of nausea, weakness and blurring of vision. Her plasma digoxin concentration is 2.8 nmol/L (2.0 ng/mL, i.e. at the top of the therapeutic range) and her potassium is 2.7 mmol/L. She is in complete heart block. (See *Cardiology*, Sections 1.3 and 2.2.1.)

Clinical approach
Although the digoxin concentration taken more than 6 h after the last dose of digoxin is not significantly elevated, the patient has symptoms of digoxin toxicity. The existence of hypokalaemia makes the diagnosis of digoxin toxicity very likely and, with correction of the plasma potassium and discontinuation of her digitalis, her symptoms resolved over

Example 20: More trouble with the foxglove (*continued*)

3 days. Her heart failure was then treated with an ACE inhibitor as well as the loop diuretic. This combination did not result in hypokalaemia and she was able to tolerate her digoxin again at a reduced dose of 187.5 µg daily.

This is an example of a dose-related toxic effect of digoxin brought about by hypokalaemia (a pharmacodynamic rather than a pharmacokinetic interaction). Digoxin binds to, and inhibits, the Na^+/K^+-ATPase and the affinity of this interaction is enhanced in the presence of a low extracellular potassium.

Dose-related anaphylactoid reaction

Example 21: Anaphylactic reaction

Case history
An 18-year-old, unemployed man is admitted to hospital 6 h after taking 60 tablets of 500 mg paracetamol. Blood is taken for a plasma paracetamol concentration and, as he has taken a significant overdose, an infusion of *N*-acetylcysteine is started. Ten minutes after the end of the loading dose of *N*-acetylcysteine, he becomes flushed, dizzy, anxious and wheezy, and his blood pressure falls to 85/62 mmHg. (See *Emergency medicine*, Section 2.1.)

Clinical approach
An anaphylactoid reaction is diagnosed and the *N*-acetylcysteine infusion is discontinued. He is treated with intravenous chlorpheniramine and hydrocortisone, and nebulized salbutamol. After a litre of saline, his blood pressure is restored to normal and he is well. His plasma paracetamol concentration is reported as 1.8 mmol/L. The *N*-acetylcysteine is restarted at the maintenance level and he remains asymptomatic and makes an uneventful recovery.

Although clinically indistinguishable from an anaphylactic reaction, this was a dose-related anaphylactoid reaction caused by a direct effect of the *N*-acetylcysteine on mast cell and basophil degranulation. Unlike an anaphylactic reaction, there is no involvement of IgE and hence it is almost always safe to restart the infusion, albeit at a dose lower than that which precipitated the problem.

4.4 Non-dose-related adverse drug reactions

Non-dose-related adverse drug reactions are unrelated to the known pharmacology of the drug and are thus difficult to predict. They arise by two main mechanisms: immunological reactions and genetic variations (Table 16).

Table 16 Examples of non-dose-related adverse drug reactions.

Genetic variation	Haemolysis caused by oxidant drugs in patients with glucose-6-phosphate dehydrogenase deficiency and some haemoglobinopathies
	Acute intermittent porphyria associated with enzyme-inducing drugs
	Methaemoglobinaemia resulting from oxidant drugs in patients with methaemoglobin reductase deficiency
	Malignant hyperpyrexia caused by suxamethonium or halothane
	Periodic paralysis precipitated by drugs that alter plasma potassium concentrations
	Glucocorticoid-induced glaucoma
Immunological reactions	Anaphylaxis caused by penicillin
	Thrombocytopenia resulting from quinine
	Acute interstitial nephritis due to penicillins
	Contact dermatitis resulting from topical creams
Pseudoallergic reactions	Ampicillin/amoxycillin rash in patients with glandular fever

Immunologically mediated adverse drug reactions

Immunologically mediated adverse drug reactions pose significant therapeutic problems. They are almost always unpredictable and often severe, and it is virtually impossible to be forewarned of the potential immunogenicity of a new drug from preclinical animal testing.

It is generally true that only molecules with a molecular weight of more than 1000 are capable of acting as immunogens, and yet most drugs are small molecules with a molecular weight of less than 500. Small molecules must therefore become covalently bound to macromolecules to be able to elicit an immune response (the hapten hypothesis of drug hypersensitivity). Almost any drug can give rise to an allergic response, but it is clear that some drugs are particularly likely to cause hypersensitivity reactions. However, even these drugs do not provoke allergic reactions in the great majority of patients, and it is likely that genetic factors play an important role in the susceptibility to drug allergy.

Patients with asthma, hayfever or eczema (so-called 'atopic' individuals) and those with hereditary angio-oedema are more at risk of developing drug allergies, particularly to penicillin.

Some drugs may conjugate to macromolecules and thus become immunogenic (e.g. penicillin, which undergoes spontaneous degradation in solution to chemically reactive products), whereas others may need to be converted enzymatically to reactive metabolites that then bind covalently to proteins (e.g. the antimalarial drug amodiaquine). The immunogenic potential of a drug is further influenced by the ability of detoxification mechanisms to clear such immunogens. Some drugs are readily converted to reactive metabolites that can bind to macromolecules, but yet are rarely immunogenic (e.g. ethinyloestradiol); this may be because the reactive metabolites or any conjugates formed are rapidly detoxified.

Immunogens may induce the formation of specific antibodies, reacting only with the parent drug compound, or they may result in the formation of antibodies that can cross-react with other antigens (e.g. autoantigens). As well as antibody-mediated effects, drugs can initiate antibody-independent T-cell-mediated reactions.

Do immune responses to drugs matter?

The formation of drug–macromolecule immunogens occurs commonly and, in the case of some drugs, probably in all recipients. Many individuals will produce an antibody response but relatively few go on to develop the full allergic drug reaction and the determinants of individual sensitivity are largely unknown. Most immune responses to drugs are not associated with the development of hypersensitivity reactions and appear to be harmless or of little importance. Sometimes antibodies directed against a drug may diminish its effect, e.g. the thrombolytic drug streptokinase is generally given in large doses because many individuals have antibodies that react with streptokinase and effectively neutralize a substantial proportion of the dose administered.

Drug hypersensitivity reactions have been classified on the basis of immunological mechanism as shown in Table 17. However, although some drugs are associated with particular types of hypersensitivity reactions, some, e.g. penicillin, may be involved with more than one type of reaction (Table 18). Furthermore, the precise clinical manifestations of drug hypersensitivity reactions can vary considerably, and strict adherence to immunological classifications is not particularly helpful in clinical practice. The following are examples that illustrate some of the possible mechanisms underlying drug hypersensitivity.

Anaphylactic reactions

Example 22: Twice bitten

Case history
A 24-year-old man is bitten by a dog and attends an A&E department where he is given co-amoxiclav. One hour after taking the first dose at home, he becomes very unwell with severe itching, wheezing and chest tightness. His GP is called and diagnoses an acute anaphylactic reaction and, in view of the patient's worsening condition, administers intramuscular epinephrine (adrenaline), intravenous hydrocortisone and chlorpheniramine, and nebulized salbutamol. The patient is

Classification	Antigen	Antibody	Effect
Type I: anaphylaxis	Free in circulation; multivalent	IgE, fixed to mast cells/basophils	Release of vasoactive and inflammatory mediators
Type II: cytotoxic	Fixed on cell membrane	Free in circulation; IgG, IgM or IgA	Antigen–antibody cross-linking, complement fixation, cell lysis
Type III: immune complex	Free in circulation in excess	Free in circulation; IgG	Immune complex deposition
Type IV: cell mediated	T killer cell interacts with antigen on cell membrane		Cell death

Table 17 The Gell and Coombs classification of hypersensitivity.

Table 18 Hypersensitivity reactions associated with penicillin.

Clinical presentation	Immunological classification
Acute anaphylaxis: urticaria, angio-oedema, hypotension, bronchospasm	Type I
Haemolytic anaemia, seen usually with high dosages and prolonged treatment	Type II
Fever, urticaria, maculopapular rash, arthritis, glomerulonephritis	Type III
Contact dermatitis from skin creams containing penicillin	Type IV

Example 22: Twice bitten (*continued*)

admitted to hospital and makes a full and rapid recovery. On further questioning, he recalls a previous less severe reaction to penicillin given for recurrent tonsillitis as a child. (See *Rheumatology and clinical immunology*, Sections 1.9 and 2.2.)

Clinical approach
Anaphylactic or type I allergic reactions occur in about 1–5 in 10 000 people treated with penicillins. The reaction is caused by antigen (the penicillin) reacting with IgE antibodies on the surface of mast cells and basophils. This results in the release of a wide range of vasoactive and inflammatory mediators including histamine, serotonin (5-HT) and leukotrienes. In the case of allergic reactions to penicillin, there is cross-allergy with cephalosporins in about 10% of cases.

 To minimize the risk of acute anaphylactic reactions, it is essential to take a full drug and allergy history from all patients. The difficulty lies in knowing how to interpret reports of rashes associated with penicillin usage. The safest thing to do is avoid penicillins if there is doubt.

Halothane hepatitis

The inhalational anaesthetic agent halothane causes a mild and transient derangement of hepatocellular

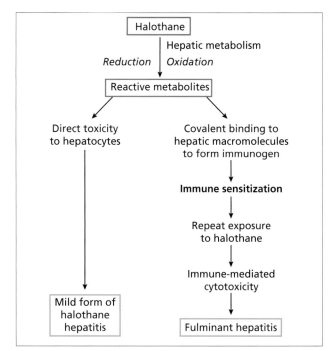

Fig. 23 The steps involved in halothane-induced liver damage.

function in up to 30% of patients. Serum transaminases are increased and liver histology may show mild focal necrotic lesions. Previous exposure to halothane is not a prerequisite for this reaction, which is caused by reactive metabolic intermediates of halothane binding directly to hepatocytes. Much more rarely (about 1 in 35 000 patients), a severe and fulminant hepatitis occurs (with a mortality rate of about 90%) and this is the result of an immunologically mediated reaction (Fig. 23).

In the liver, halothane is metabolized by reduction and oxidation. The reduced metabolites react directly with hepatocytes and are responsible for the mild hepatic disturbance. Halothane is oxidized, by a hepatic cytochrome P450 enzyme to trifluoroacetyl chloride, which can covalently bind to hepatic macromolecules and become antigenic. When this occurs, if the patient has a further general anaesthetic containing halothane, immune-mediated cytotoxicity may result in progression to fulminant hepatitis.

 As might be anticipated in a hypersensitivity reaction, the incidence of fulminant hepatitis increases after multiple exposures to halothane, and repeated use within 3 months should be avoided. It is also advisable to avoid the use of halothane in any patient with previously unexplained postoperative jaundice.

Immune haemolytic anaemias

 Drugs can give rise to haemolysis by direct chemical means (e.g. the action of oxidant drugs in glucose-6-phosphate dehydrogenase deficiency) or immune-mediated red cell destruction. For immune haemolysis to occur, antibodies or complement must be bound to the red cell and this can arise by three main mechanisms (Table 19).

Table 19 Drugs that most commonly cause immune haemolytic anaemia.

Mechanism of haemolysis	Drug	Antibody
Covalent binding of drug to red cell membranes	Penicillin, cephalosporins	IgG
Immune complex association with red cell membranes and subsequent fixation of complement	Quinine, quinidine, sulphonamides, isoniazid, rifampicin	IgM
Autoantibodies that recognize red cell components	Methyldopa, levodopa, mefenamic acid	IgG

DIRECT BINDING OF THE DRUG TO THE RED CELL MEMBRANE

When penicillin is used in high doses for a prolonged period of time, the drug binds covalently to red cell membranes and this hapten–membrane complex may then elicit an immune response, with the production of specific, mainly IgG, antibodies. Antigen–antibody crosslinking occurs and extravascular haemolysis results. When the drug is discontinued, the haemolysis resolves but may recur on second exposure. Cephalosporins can cross react with these antibodies and cause similar effects.

IMMUNE COMPLEX FORMATION

In this form of haemolysis, covalent binding of drugs or their metabolites to circulating free proteins is thought to give rise to antibodies, mainly of the IgM type. In the presence of the drug, antigen–antibody complexes can then associate with red cell membranes, complement is activated and profound intravascular haemolysis occurs.

Haemolysis does not occur with the first dose of drug, but on second or subsequent exposure, and it resolves promptly on withdrawing the drug.

AUTOANTIBODY FORMATION

Certain drugs (methyldopa, levodopa and mefenamic acid), when given over a long period of time, can give rise to the formation of IgG antibodies which cross react with components in the red cell membrane and cause extravascular haemolysis. This is rarely severe and ceases when the drug is withdrawn.

Genetic variations

Glucose-6-phosphate dehydrogenase deficiency

 Glucose-6-phosphate dehydrogenase (G6PD) deficiency is the most common human enzymopathy, affecting over 10 million people worldwide. Several hundred biochemically or genetically different forms of the enzyme have been identified, but in essence the condition arises from reduced enzymatic activity of G6PD, which results, in severe cases, in red cells being more susceptible to damage from oxidizing agents.

G6PD is an enzyme that generates NADPH, the reduced form of nicotinamide adenine dinucleotide phosphate (NADP), from NADP (see *Biochemistry and metabolism*, Section 2). NADPH is required to convert oxidized glutathione to the reduced form, and it is this reduced glutathione that protects erythrocytes from damage from oxidizing agents (Fig. 24). Certain drugs act as oxidants and may precipitate haemolysis in patients who are deficient in G6PD (Table 20). The most severe forms of G6PD deficiency are seen in individuals in whom enzyme activity is below 5% of normal. Less severe forms, in which enzyme activity is between 10% and 30% of normal, usually become apparent only when affected

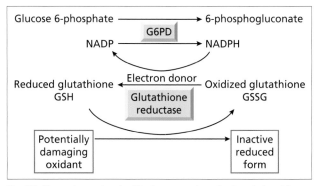

Fig. 24 The pathways involved in the generation of reduced glutathione in red cells.

Table 20 Oxidant drugs which can precipitate haemolysis in patients with G6PD deficiency.

Drug class	Common examples
Analgesics	Aspirin
Antbiotics	Chloramphenicol
	Nitrofurantoin
	Sulphonamides
Antimalarials	Primaquine
	Dapsone
	Quinine
Miscellaneous	Quinidine, vitamin K

Table 21 Some of the more commonly prescribed drugs which have been reported to precipitate an attack of acute porphyria.

Drug class	Common examples
Antibiotics	Sulphonamides, tetracycline, isoniazid, griseofulvin, nitrofurantoin, rifampicin
Anticonvulsants	Phenytoin, carbamazepine, ethosuximide, primidone
Oral hypoglycaemic agents	Tolbutamide, chlorpropamide
Sedatives/hypnotics	Chlordiazepoxide, nitrazepam, oxazepam, barbiturates
Sex steroids	Oral contraceptives, oestrogens
Miscellaneous	Ethanol, imipramine, methyldopa

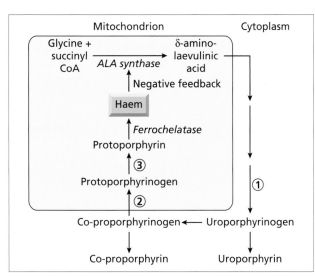

Fig. 25 The pathways involved in porphyrin and haem biosynthesis: (1) the enzymatic step involving uroporphyrinogen I synthase and uroporphyrinogen co-synthetase, which is affected in acute intermittent porphyria; (2) the reaction involving co-proporphyrinogen oxidase, which is deficient in hereditary co-proporphyria; (3) the reaction catalysed by protoporphyrinogen oxidase, which is deficient in variegate porphyria.

individuals are treated with those drugs that have the greatest potential action as oxidizing agents.

Acute porphyria

The acute porphyrias are a group of genetically determined metabolic disorders characterized by defects in the enzymes associated with porphyrin and haem biosynthesis. In all of the various types, there is increased activity of the rate-limiting enzyme δ-aminolaevulinic acid (ALA) synthase; the different forms are characterized by specific enzyme defects further along the pathway of porphyrin synthesis (Fig. 25). (See *Biochemistry and metabolism*, Section 6.)

Acute intermittent porphyria, hereditary co-proporphyria and variegate porphyria can all present acutely with abdominal and neuropsychiatric symptoms. In hereditary co-proporphyria and variegate porphyria, there may also be skin photosensitivity. Patients with a genetic predisposition to acute porphyria may develop an acute attack after exposure to alcohol or certain drugs, which in general are inducers of hepatic mono-oxygenase enzymes (Table 21).

The way in which accumulation of porphyrins causes symptoms is not clear. Porphyrins are known to be photosensitizing agents and the cutaneous manifestations of the porphyrias may be the result of damage from photochemical reactions arising as a result of the absorption by porphyrins of radiant energy in the ultraviolet region of the spectrum. The abdominal and neuropsychiatric manifestations of the disease are not so readily explained.

Chapel H, Haeney M, Misbah S, Snowden N. *Essentials of Clinical Immunology*, 4th edn. Oxford: Blackwell Science, 1999.
Journal of Hepatology 1997; 26 (suppl 2) is devoted to drugs and the liver.
Pirohamed M, Madden S, Park BK. Idiosyncratic drug reactions. Metabolic bioactivation as a pathogenic mechanism. *Clin Pharmacokinet* 1996; 31: 215–30.

4.5 Adverse reactions caused by long-term effects of drugs

When drugs are taken over a long period of time, there may be problems of cumulative toxicity. Recognizing this sort of gradual drug toxicity is more difficult than many of the reactions described so far, because the index of suspicion for adverse drug reactions is often low when the drug concerned has been taken for a long time. Drugs can also cause adaptive changes that may predispose to long-term adverse effects and withdrawal syndromes if they are discontinued abruptly.

Cumulative drug toxicity

Amiodarone

Example 23: It seemed useful at the time

Case history
A 59-year-old man with troublesome paroxysmal atrial fibrillation and normal left ventricular function is treated with amiodarone with useful suppression of symptoms. Three years later he re-presents with progressive breathlessness and his GP finds that he has widespread fine crepitations in both lung fields. A chest radiograph and computed tomography (CT) scan show that he has diffuse interstitial infiltrates. A CT cut through the liver demonstrates high-signal intensity (Fig. 26). The diagnosis of amiodarone lung was made, the drug was discontinued and he was treated with high-dose steroids. (See *Respiratory medicine*, Sections 1.4 and 2.8.5.)

Clinical approach
The antiarrhythmic drug amiodarone is very lipophilic and highly tissue bound, with an elimination half-life in the order of 45–60 days. Gradual tissue accumulation of amiodarone and its principal metabolite desethylamiodarone is associated with deposition of lipofuscin in the organs in which long-term toxic effects are most commonly seen. However, the relationship between lipofuscin deposition and the adverse effects of amiodarone is not absolute, because many patients will accumulate lipofuscin but not have evidence of adverse effects.

Lithium

Lithium is widely used in the long-term treatment of bipolar affective disorder; about 5% of patients develop a benign diffuse enlargement of the thyroid gland. Lithium interferes with the iodination of tyrosine, and as a result thyroxine output from the thyroid falls. Most patients taking lithium long term are euthyroid, because there is a compensatory rise in thyroid-stimulating hormone (TSH) release from the pituitary. It is this rise in TSH that causes the diffuse enlargement of the thyroid gland and, if it is troublesome, it can be treated with thyroxine, which suppresses TSH production.

Chloroquine

The antimalarial drug chloroquine can cause a lichenoid skin eruption when used long term but is otherwise quite well tolerated in the dosages used for the prophylaxis of malaria. Chloroquine also has a place in the treatment of connective tissue diseases, such as rheumatoid arthritis, and lupus erythematosus; in these conditions it may be used in substantially higher doses than in malaria prophylaxis. Under these circumstances, irreversible retinopathy is a serious adverse effect and is related to the high affinity

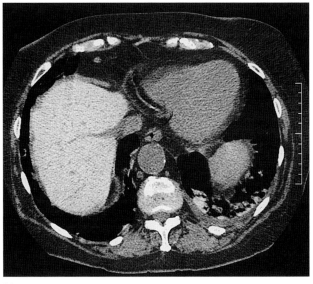

(a)

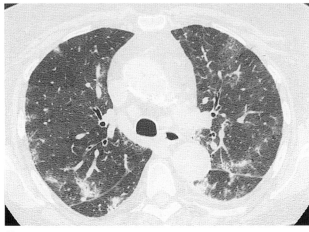

(b)

Fig. 26 (a) CT scan of the liver. The liver is hyperdense (118 Hounsfield units or HU) and the consolidation in the left lower lobe is also hyperdense (131 HU). Both of these characteristics are typical of iodine deposition and the combination is pathognomonic of amiodarone accumulation. (b) High-resolution CT scan of the lung: bilateral peripheral ground-glass change with interstitial fibrosis. (By kind permission of Dr N. Moore.)

of chloroquine for melanin, which results in its accumulation in retinal pigment. Regular ophthalmological examination to detect early subclinical changes in retinal function is essential to avoid progressive visual loss in patients on high-dose chloroquine.

Withdrawal reactions

Long-term treatment with some drugs causes adaptive changes in homeostatic mechanisms or induces a state of drug dependence, so that when the drug is abruptly discontinued a withdrawal reaction occurs. Perhaps the most commonly encountered withdrawal syndrome is that of delirium tremens. Benzodiazepines, opioid analgesics and barbiturates are all associated with specific syndromes, which may arise on sudden discontinuation of therapy (or abuse).

Example 24: Don't stop taking the pills

Case history
A 73-year-old man developed nausea, vomiting and diarrhoea. His GP diagnosed food poisoning and advised that he went to bed and took plenty of fluids; 3 days later he was worse and was admitted to hospital, where he was found to be severely dehydrated, hypotensive and in acute renal failure. It transpired that, because of the vomiting he had felt unable to take his usual tablets, which included prednisolone 10 mg a day, prescribed for temporal arteritis 18 months earlier. (See *Emergency medicine*, Section 1.20 and *Endocrinology*, Section 2.2.2.)

Clinical approach
This patient became dehydrated because of his diarrhoea and vomiting, but the problem was compounded by abrupt steroid withdrawal leading to Addisonian crisis. He made a good recovery with fluid and steroid replacement, and was given advice about what to do in the future if he became unwell.

Long-term corticosteroid therapy is associated with suppression of the hypothalamic–pituitary–adrenal axis. If steroid therapy is withdrawn, adrenal insufficiency may occur either acutely or at a later stage when heightened physical stress occurs (e.g. infection or major surgery).

4.6 Adverse reactions caused by delayed effects of drugs

Some drugs have been appropriately called 'wonder drugs' inasmuch as one wonders what they will do next.
(Samuel E. Stumpf)

When adverse reactions occur months or years after a drug has been discontinued, it is extremely difficult to identify a causal relationship. Drug-induced neoplasia is a particular concern because it is often not apparent for many years after the introduction of a drug and it may not have been anticipated in preclinical toxicological testing in animals.

A high proportion of patients receiving immunosuppressive therapy after organ transplantation develop malignant lymphomas (up to 20% in some series). It seems likely that this is as a result of the depression of the protective immune response, rather than any direct carcinogenic effect of immunosuppressive drugs. However, the risks of lymphoma in this group of patients are usually more than balanced by the severity of the illness for which transplantation was initially performed.

In the early 1970s, there were several reports of a very rare tumour (vaginal adenocarcinoma) in young girls whose mothers had been given oestrogens (diethylstilboestrol) during the first trimester of pregnancy for the treatment of uterine bleeding. The spontaneous incidence of this tumour in girls whose mothers have not received diethylstilboestrol is so low that it was relatively easy to make a direct association with the drug in new cases.

Chronic overuse of analgesic drugs, particularly those containing phenacetin, causes renal papillary necrosis and ultimately renal failure. In addition, there is an association between long-term phenacetin abuse and transitional cell carcinomas of the renal tract. Although phenacetin is no longer marketed, transitional cell tumours still arise as a late complication of its use.

4.7 Teratogenic effects

Many drugs have the potential to damage the fetus during pregnancy—always consult the data sheet for any drug that you intend to use in women of child-bearing age.

See Section 5.3, page 73.

5 Prescribing in special circumstances

> *I do not want two diseases—one nature made, one doctor made. (Napoleon Bonaparte, 1820)*

5.1 Introduction

Some specific patient groups merit special consideration when prescribing medication. The altered physiology of pregnancy and pathophysiology of renal or hepatic disease can significantly change pharmacokinetic and pharmacodynamic responses. Such conditions are further sources of variation in drug response between individuals (Fig. 27). In the pregnant patient, the developing fetus may be exposed to drugs by transplacental transfer, and the breast-feeding mother may inadvertently expose the neonate to drugs in breast milk. In such patients, we need to be even more careful than usual before we put pen to drug chart.

- Hepatic disease
- Renal disease
- Pregnancy
- Pharmacogenetics
- Drug interactions
- Age

↓

- Altered pharmacokinetics
- Altered pharmacodynamics

↓

- Unexpected toxicity
- Unexpected therapeutic failure

Fig. 27 Some examples of sources of between-subject variability in both pharmacokinetic and pharmacodynamic responses.

5.2 Prescribing and liver disease

Example 25: A man with a failing liver

Case history
A medical opinion is sought on a 46-year-old man who was admitted 5 days previously with abdominal pain. When admitted he was unkempt, smelling of alcohol, and aggressive and abusive to the nursing staff. He was icteric and had abnormal liver function tests. He was managed

Example 25: A man with a failing liver (*continued*)

conservatively. His conscious level has deteriorated markedly over the last 24 h. (See *Gastroenterology and hepatology*, Sections 1.7, 1.16, 2.9 and 2.10.)

Clinical approach
You are going to need to go through the full assessment and consideration of the causes of deteriorating conscious level (see *Emergency medicine*, Section 1.26). Of special consideration is the possibility of a drug-induced deterioration which has arisen because insufficient account has been taken of the effects of impaired liver function. Clinical assessment therefore requires full consideration of clinical and laboratory markers of liver disease seen in the context of his recent inpatient medication.

The hospital notes should be reviewed for previous admissions with alcoholic or other liver disease. The patient's family or GP might shed light on his premorbid state. Look carefully for stigmata of chronic liver disease, which suggest a significant metabolic problem. Look for signs of sedative drug effects, such as pinpoint pupils or respiratory depression from opiates. His liver function tests are deranged; take particular note of the clotting screen and serum albumin as indices of biosynthetic capacity. Check renal function, impairment of which will compromise other routes of drug clearance.

Review the drug and fluid balance chart in detail. The likely scenario is one of sedation as a result of a combination of regular opioid analgesia for his presenting complaint of abdominal pain together with benzodiazepines to control his agitated confusion, which may be related to alcohol withdrawal. Although excessive doses may not have been employed, these drugs may have gradually accumulated to marked sedative levels, an effect exacerbated if there is coexisting renal impairment.

When assessing a patient, always consider the possibility that the patient's clinical state may be at least in part drug induced. Always carefully review all prescribing information, both drug and total dose administered, especially if the patient falls into one of the 'special circumstances' discussed in this section.

General considerations

The liver performs many important metabolic functions. In the presence of significant hepatic dysfunction there may be altered pharmacodynamic responses to drugs and there are frequently clinically important changes in the pharmacokinetics of drugs which make prescribing in liver disease potentially hazardous (Table 22).

71

Table 22 Liver disease may result in hepatocellular dysfunction, cholestasis and portosystemic shunting of blood. Such dysfunction results in altered pharmacokinetics and pharmacodynamics of many drugs. Some common examples are shown to illustrate the effects of such pathophysiology.

Drug	Reason for concern
Morphine	Impaired metabolism may lead to accumulation and risk of coma
	Increased CNS sensitivity may result in precipitation of encephalopathy
Diuretics	Can precipitate encephalopathy due to excessive potassium loss
Oral anticoagulants	Enhanced response due to reduced absorption of vitamin K in obstructive jaundice and reduced production of vitamin K-dependent clotting factors
Oral antidiabetic agents	Increased risk of hypoglycaemia with sulphonylureas
	Increased risk of lactic acidosis with biguanides
Theophylline	Impaired metabolism and risk of toxicity with therapeutic dose
Chlormethiazole	Marked CNS and respiratory depression due to increased sensitivity and impaired metabolism
Phenytoin	Increased risk of CNS toxicity due to reduced metabolism, especially if associated renal impairment
Lignocaine	Risk of severe CNS toxicity due to impaired metabolism and narrow therapeutic index
Vitamin D	Impaired hepatic hydroxylation of vitamin D Calcifediol (25 hydroxy vitamin D3 is preferred)
Corticosteroids	Reduced protein binding results in increased sensitivity to steroids
	Risk of causing fluid overload
Non-steroidal anti-inflammatory drugs	Risk of fluid overload
Carbenoxolone	Risk of fluid overload
Rifampicin	Excreted unchanged in bile; may accumulate in obstructive jaundice

Hepatocellular dysfunction gives rise to:
- impaired drug detoxification
- abnormal brain sensitivity
- altered coagulation
- low serum albumin and altered drug binding
- risk of fluid overload.

The effect of liver disease on drug handling is not always predictable and depends on the aetiology of the disease, the stage of the illness and the degree of functional impairment. The last is difficult to predict from routinely monitored 'liver function tests' alone. As with all adverse drug reactions, problems are most likely to arise when dealing with drugs that have a narrow therapeutic ratio and are heavily dependent on hepatic metabolism, especially if other mechanisms of clearance are impaired.

Remember that patients with liver disease often have associated:
- renal impairment
- cardiac impairment
- poor nutrition
- acute and chronic alcohol abuse
- intravenous drug abuse
- multiple drug therapy.

In liver disease cholestasis may be associated with:
- failure of biliary drug excretion
- malabsorption of vitamins and drugs.

In liver disease portosystemic shunts give rise to:
- reduced first-pass drug metabolism
- increased risk of gastrointestinal bleeding
- enhanced risk of hepatic encephalopathy.

Assessment of the degree of liver dysfunction

It is difficult to make an accurate clinical assessment of the metabolic capacity of the liver, and thus adjust the dosage of a drug in proportion to the changes in distribution, metabolism and pharmacodynamic responses. This results partly from the following factors:
- Hepatic function can fluctuate greatly over time
- The liver has great reserve capacity
- There is considerable interindividual variation in hepatic drug metabolism
- Conventional liver function tests (alanine transaminase (ALT), alkaline phosphatase (ALP), γ-glutamyl transferase (γGT)) are markers of liver cell damage rather than metabolic function.

Adjustment of drug dosage in liver disease

Unlike in renal disease, there is no simple test of liver function that enables a therapeutic regimen to be simply adjusted. The following increase the likelihood of abnormal drug handling:
- encephalopathy
- ascites
- abnormal coagulation
- low serum albumin
- jaundice.

Susceptibility of patients with liver disease to known hepatotoxic drugs

Some drugs carry risks of causing hepatic damage (Table 23). This is mainly because of the following:
- Liver disease may increase the risk of some idiosyncratic hypersensitivity-type reactions
- Liver disease significantly increases the risk of dose-related reactions.

Table 23 Drug-induced liver damage may occur rarely and unpredictably at low doses (idiosyncratic) or be a common manifestation of prolonged high-dose administration (dose dependent). The damage resulting will be predominantly liver cell damage (hepatocellular) or predominantly interference with metabolism and excretion of bilirubin (cholestatic).

	Idiosyncractic	Dose dependent
Hepatocellular	General anaesthetics: • Halothane Antidepressants: • Monoamine oxidase inhibitors Antiepileptics: • Carbamazepine • Phenytoin • Phenobarbitone • Sodium valproate Antimicrobials: • Sulphonamides • Isoniazid Antihypertensives: • Methyldopa • Hydralazine	Alcohol Paracetamol Amiodarone Ketoconazole
Cholestatic	Phenothiazine neuroleptics: • Chlorpromazine Sulphonylureas: • Glibenclamide • Chlorpropamide • Tolbutamide Carbimazole	Sex steroids: • Methyltestosterone • Anabolic steroids • Synthetic oestrogens • Synthetic progestagens Antimicrobials: • Fusidic acid • Rifampicin • Erythromycin

Potentially hepatotoxic drugs should be avoided, or (if absolutely necessary) used in reduced dosage in patients with pre-existing liver disease because they may cause further damage to the reduced hepatic reserve; they may also confuse the management of the existing liver disease.

Drugs are frequently implicated in the aetiology of both common and rare forms of hepatic disease. Always consider the possibility of drug-induced liver disease if there are unexplained abnormalities in the routine 'liver function tests'.

General principles of prescribing in liver disease

When prescribing for patients with liver disease bear in mind the following:
• Always perform a careful risk–benefit assessment; if benefits do not outweigh the risks then do not prescribe
• Select drugs with no potential for hepatotoxicity
• Select drugs that are mainly excreted unchanged by the kidneys
• Avoid drugs with effects on the CNS
• Avoid drugs that affect coagulation
• Avoid drugs that promote salt and water retention
• Start with small doses and increase cautiously
• Monitor levels of drug when feasible.

British National Formulary, Appendix II.
James I. Prescribing in liver disease. *Br J Hosp Med* 1975; 13 (suppl 1): 67–76.
Rodighiero V. Effects of liver disease on pharmacokinetics. An update. *Clin Pharmacokinet* 1999; 37: 399–431.

5.3 Prescribing in pregnancy

Drugs may be administered to pregnant women, if required, from the fourth to seventh month of gestation.
(Hippocrates, 400 BC)

General principles of prescribing in pregnancy

• Remember that, although medication often has to be prescribed, 'no drug is safe beyond all doubt in early pregnancy' (*British National Formulary*).
• Safety data are generally derived from a retrospective analysis of accumulated patient exposure (controlled clinical trials would be unethical in such circumstances), hence older drugs with better known side effects are generally preferred.
• During pregnancy the mother and baby constitute a single 'maternofetal unit'—the well-being of the mother is an absolute requirement for the well-being of the fetus.
• The mother should always be treated to maintain optimal health while all attempts are made to reduce the risk to the fetus (Fig. 28).

Example 26: Deep venous thrombosis in pregnancy

Case history
A 20-year-old woman presents at 10 weeks into her pregnancy with a painful swollen calf. (See *Cardiology*, Sections 1.9 and 2.18.)

Clinical approach
Your main concern is that the patient has developed a deep venous thrombosis (DVT) in the context of pregnancy and will thus require anticoagulation. The management of any medical condition in a pregnant woman is complicated by the potential harm of any prescribed drugs to the fetus, together with alteration in maternal drug handling as a consequence of the physiological changes of pregnancy. Warfarin and heparin both have particular problems associated with their use in pregnancy (Tables 24 and 25 and Fig. 29). In addition to the usual bleeding risk to the mother associated with anticoagulation, warfarin readily crosses the placenta, enters the fetal circulation and poses a serious risk to the fetus. Heparin (both fractionated and unfractionated) is a highly charged compound with high molecular weight; it is thus unusual in that it does not cross the placenta. The use of heparin in pregnancy is associated with minimal risk to the fetus, but is associated with increased maternal risk. However, the fetotoxicity associated with warfarin leads most obstetricians to prefer regimens based on heparin alone. (Fig. 29, Regimen 2)

Timing (weeks)	Stage	Events	Potential toxicity	Comments
2	Blastogenesis	Conception to implantation Establishment utero-placental perfusion	'All or none period' Fetus survives unharmed or early death and spontaneous abortion	Small number of pluripotent cells replace damaged cells or all cells damaged and fetus aborted Mother may experience 'late period'
4 6 8	Embryogenesis	Organogenesis and development of all major systems	Drug-induced fetal mal-formations	Many women still unaware that they are pregnant
38	Fetogenesis	Further growth and differentiation of major systems, esp. central nervous system	Growth retardation Intellectual impairment	Subtle effects on cognition may go undetected

Fig. 28 The risk of drug toxicity is intimately related to the stages of fetal development.

Table 24 Fetal complications of warfarin therapy.

Complication	Time of exposure	Manifestations	Aetiology
Warfarin embryopathy	'Critical window' of 6–9 weeks of pregnancy	Nasal hypoplasia, depression of nasal bridge, hypoplasia of extremities, stippling of epiphyses	Reduced carboxylation of calcium-binding proteins
Neurological damage	After critical window	Mental retardation, microcephaly, optic atrophy and blindness	Possibly haemorrhagic in origin, hence may be reduced by tight anticoagulant control
Haemorrhagic	During delivery	Traumatic intracranial haemorrhage during vaginal delivery	Reduced clotting factors in full-term neonate compared with older infants

Table 25 Maternal complications of heparin therapy.

Complication	Comment
Osteoporosis	Subclinical bone demineralization common Significant demineralization with fractures is rare
Immune thrombocytopenia	Very rare
Maternal haemorrhage at time of delivery	Risk reduced by good anticoagulant control

Complications of prescribing during pregnancy

Drug treatment in the pregnant woman raises issues related to both the well-being of the mother and the well-being of the fetus.

Fetal well-being

The main concern relates to possible transplacental transfer of drugs (Fig. 28). In general the following rules apply:

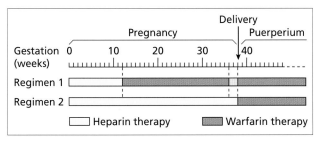

Fig. 29 Anticoagulant regimens in pregnancy.

• All drugs cross the placenta unless extremely large and highly polar (e.g. heparin).

• The degree and rate of transfer are fastest for small, non-polar, lipid-soluble drugs.

• After a single dose of drug, the fetus is generally exposed to a lower concentration of drug than the mother, and the time taken to achieve a peak concentration in the fetus is delayed.

• After repeat dosing, the fetus is generally exposed to similar steady-state concentrations as the mother.

• The nature of any fetal damage depends on the time of drug administration in relation to stage of fetal development.

Teratogenicity

A teratogen (Greek: *teras*, monster) is a substance that causes structural or functional abnormalities in a fetus exposed to the substance (Table 26). In general, the following comments apply to teratogenicity:

• It is associated with a window of opportunity related to critical developmental activities in the target system(s), e.g. warfarin teratogenicity between 6 and 9 weeks of development.

• It is a dose-dependent effect.

• It is species dependent (may be non-teratogenic in some species, or affect a different system).

• The mechanism is often obscure but may be the result of specific or multifactorial effects on the embryo, or effects on the placenta or the mother.

• The susceptibility is influenced by the genetic profile of the fetus.

• Many abnormalities that are attributed to drug treatment occur with a background frequency in the absence of the drug.

• Many disease states in pregnancy are themselves 'teratogenic'.

All prescribing decisions have to be carefully assessed in pregnancy, but there are some circumstances that commonly cause difficulties:
• Chronic medical problems existing before pregnancy, e.g. asthma, epilepsy
• Medical emergencies in a previously fit mother that arise during the pregnancy, e.g. thromboembolic disease, cardiac dysrhythmias, pre-eclampsia, infections
• Minor ailments related or unrelated to the pregnancy, e.g. nausea, back pain.

Table 26 Commonly prescribed drugs that are fetotoxic. Some drugs, such as ACE inhibitors, should not be prescribed whereas others, such as carbamazepine, are commonly used with close monitoring.

Drug or class	Adverse effect	Comments
Aminoglycoside antibiotics	Ototoxicity	For example, gentamicin
Carbamazepine	Increased risk of neural tube defects	About 1% of pregnancies. Supplementation with folic acid prior to and during pregnancy, close monitoring by AFP and ultrasonography
ACE inhibitors Angiotensin receptor antagonists	Renal agenesis and oligohydramnions	Angiotensin is important in controlling development of the fetal kidney
Coumarin anticoagulants, e.g. warfarin	Fetal warfarin syndrome of CNS and skeletal abnormalities	About 16% of fetuses affected, spontaneous abortion common (8%). Also increased risk of bleeding at term
Lithium	Increased risk of Ebstein's anomaly	Risk not known but small. Advise close ultrasound monitoring of pregnancy
Phenytoin	Fetal hydantoin syndrome with dysmorphism, CNS and skeletal defects	5–10% have full syndrome, more have partial or intellectual impairment. Alternative agent preferred, if required for seizure control then aim for low therapeutic level and close monitoring by ultrasound scanning
Tetracycline	Staining of teeth	50% incidence if exposed after 4 weeks
Valproic acid	Spina bifida, CNS and cardiac defects	About 1% risk of neural tube defects. Monitor AFP and ultrasound scanning

ACE, angiotensin-converting enzyme; AFP, alpha-fetoprotein; CNS, central nervous system.

Drug	Change in therapeutic effect	Mechanism	Comments
Lithium	Reduced	Increased renal clearance	Clearance doubles during pregnancy and significant dose increases may be required. Levels can rise rapidly after delivery if dose not reduced to prepregnancy levels
Digoxin	Reduced	Increased renal clearance	May require twice non-pregnant dose towards end of pregnancy
Phenytoin	Variable	Increased hepatic metabolism, reduced absorption, reduced plasma protein binding	Reduced plasma protein binding offsets the reduction in absorption and increase in metabolism
Penicillins	Reduced	Increased renal clearance	Half the expected plasma levels may be obtained at end of pregnancy

Table 27 Changes in physiology as a result of pregnancy can alter drug handling. This can be significant for a few common drugs and necessitate changes in dose during pregnancy.

 Human teratogens are readily identified if they frequently cause dramatic but otherwise rare malformations (e.g. thalidomide). Even drugs that are currently considered 'safe' during fetogenesis might cause very subtle effects, e.g. on cognition, that are likely to go undetected.

Complications of drug administration at term

Drugs given around the time of delivery may cause problems that arise because of one of the following:
- Interference with the progress of labour.
- Suppression of fetal systems after delivery, e.g. opioids causing respiratory depression.
- Interference with cardiopulmonary physiological changes at term, e.g. premature closure of the ductus arteriosus.
- Increased fetal and maternal bleeding during labour, e.g. warfarin.

Maternal well-being

The changes that occur in maternal physiology during pregnancy result in changes in drug handling by the body (pharmacokinetics). In general (but not always) these tend to reduce the plasma levels of active drug compared with in the non-pregnant state. Alterations in the pharmacokinetics of drugs in pregnancy can lead to unexpected toxicity or therapeutic failure at doses used in non-pregnant women. It is particularly important to monitor plasma levels of those compounds with a narrow therapeutic window whenever possible, e.g. digoxin and lithium (Table 27).

 Alterations in maternal drug handling may arise because of a number of physiological changes that occur in pregnancy:
- increased volume of distribution as a result of increase in total body water
- altered drug absorption
- reduced plasma protein binding
- increased hepatic drug metabolism
- increased renal clearance.

 The restoration of non-pregnant physiology after delivery can result in a rapid accumulation of drugs, the dose of which has been increased to maintain adequate levels towards the end of pregnancy. Early restoration of the pre-pregnancy dose is required to prevent digoxin or lithium toxicity in the puerperium.

5.4 Prescribing for women of child-bearing potential

You should remember that any woman of child-bearing potential may be pregnant (and unaware of the fact) or may become pregnant subsequently.

When prescribing for any woman of child-bearing potential it is important to:
• exclude pregnancy if prescribing a drug that might pose a known teratogenic risk
• determine whether the patient is attempting to become pregnant or at risk of an unplanned pregnancy
• consider whether the prescribed drug might interfere with hormonal methods of contraception.
  Before prescribing:
• check if the drug can cause fetal damage
• clearly inform the patient of the potential risks of using or withholding such a drug, so that she can make informed decisions regarding treatment and pregnancy.

British National Formulary, Appendix 4.
Greaves M. Anticoagulants in pregnancy. *Pharmacol Ther* 1993; 59: 311–27.
National Teratology Information Service (Regional Drug and Therapeutics Centre, Newcastle) provides telephone advice on 0191 23215253.
Prescribing in pregnancy. A series of articles published in the *British Medical Journal* covering all management of disease in all major specialties in the context of pregnancy, between December 1986 and March 1987.
Rubin P. Prescribing in pregnancy. *Practitioner* 1990; 234: 556–60.

5.5 Prescribing to lactating mothers

Example 27: Breast is best, but there can be problems

Case history
A 32-year-old nurse needed treatment for pregnancy-induced hypertension with methyldopa. This is her second child and the previous pregnancy was complicated by quite severe postnatal depression. Her blood pressure remains elevated post delivery and it is considered that she should stay on treatment. She intends to breast-feed and is concerned about passing any medication on to her baby.

Clinical approach
As with prescribing in pregnancy, most information on safety of drugs in breast-feeding relates to older agents. Most drugs are passed to some extent into breast milk and thence to the neonate, but usually this does not constitute a significant problem. It would be possible to continue methyldopa therapy because this is present in breast milk in amounts that are too small to be harmful. However, methyldopa is known to cause sedation and to increase the likelihood of a depressive episode, and given the history of severe postnatal depression continued use of this agent would not be advisable.

Example 27: Breast is best, but there can be problems (*continued*)

Most of the more modern antihypertensives are excreted to a variable extent in breast milk and the manufacturers generally advise against their use in the breast-feeding mother. However, the mother can be reassured that satisfactory management of her hypertension can be achieved without the necessity of stopping breast-feeding, and a suitable agent can be selected after discussion with the mother and reference to published advice regarding the safety of drugs in breast-feeding.

General considerations

In general, all drugs given to a breast-feeding mother will enter her breast milk, but most drugs are not selectively excreted in breast milk and hence exposure to the neonate will usually be considerably below that of the mother. However, certain drugs may be concentrated in specific organs and exaggerated pharmacokinetic or pharmacodynamic responses may be seen as a result of differences in fetal physiology, especially in pre-term babies (Table 28).

Drugs administered to the mother may suppress lactation and mothers must be fully informed of any risk to their likely ability to continue to breast-feed. Drugs that cause sedation in the adult may do so in the neonate and this may impair suckling.

Classification of drugs administered to the breast-feeding mother

In broad terms, drugs that might be used in breast-feeding mothers may be divided into three categories as follows:
1 Drugs that are known to produce specific problems and are contraindicated or should be used only with caution. If such agents are required for maternal well-being, then the mother will almost certainly need to bottle-feed (Table 29).

Table 28 The neonate may show increased sensitivity to drugs excreted in breast milk as a result of altered phamacokinetics or pharmacodynamics.

Change	Mechanism	Effect
Pharmacokinetic	Absorption	Generally unaffected
	Hepatic metabolism	Reduced albumin biosynthesis
		Reduced clotting factor synthesis
		Reduced enzymic drug metabolism
	Renal excretion	Relatively low GFR
Pharmacodynamic	—	Increased sensitivity to respiratory depressant action of morphine

GFR, glomerular filtration rate.

Table 29 A number of drugs are associated with problems in mothers who are breast-feeding and should be avoided.

Drug	Comments
Cytotoxics	Inherent toxicity
Radio-iodine	Concentrated in the milk with a milk plasma ratio of 70 : 1
	Further concentrated in the fetal thyroid gland
	Subsequent increase in risk of permanent hypothyroidism and thyroid cancer
Bromocriptine	Suppresses lactation
Chloramphenicol	Aplastic anaemia (grey baby syndrome) due to low glucuronyl transferase activity
Aspirin	Association with Reye's syndrome
Dothiepin	Sedation and respiratory depression due to active metabolite
Laxatives	Increased gastric motility and diarrhoea
Antipsychotics	Animal studies suggest potential adverse effects on development of the CNS
Antiepileptics	Some agents may cause sedation
Theophylline	Slow clearance with irritability and possible sleep disturbance

2 Drugs that can be administered because they appear in amounts in the milk that are too small to be harmful to the neonate.

3 Drugs that are not known to be harmful to the neonate, although they are present in significant quantities in breast milk.

For most drugs there is inadequate evidence to provide reliable guidance on the safety of a drug in breast-feeding. As with pregnancy, it is best to administer only those drugs that are considered necessary for maternal well-being.

British National Formulary, Appendix 5.

5.6 Prescribing in renal disease

Example 28: Doing well, but then 'went off'

Case history
You are contacted by a house officer who is getting to know her new patients; she is alarmed by the state of a 70-year-old woman who has been an inpatient for 3 weeks on an outlying ward following repair of a fractured neck of femur. Initially she did well postoperatively, apart from an episode of apparent heart failure. However, she has gradually become unwell, with confusion and drowsiness. Her renal function, last checked 2 weeks ago, showed a creatinine of 180 μmol/L and a urea of 15 mmol/L; her blood tests today reveal a creatinine of 700 μmol/L and a urea of 52 mmol/L. The house

Example 28: Doing well, but then 'went off' (*continued*)

officer attributes the deterioration to adverse effects of drugs, these being shown in Table 30. (See *Nephrology*, section 1.7.)

Table 30 Drugs prescribed before and continued during admission.

	Drug	Dosage
Drugs prescribed before and continued during admission	Furosemide (frusemide)	80 mg od (recently increased from 40 mg)
	Quinine sulphate	300 mg nocte
	Naproxen	500 mg bid
	Co-danthramer	10 mL bid
Additional drugs prescribed during admission	Lisinopril	10 mg od
	Co-codamol	2 tabs qds
	Prochlorperazine	10 mg tds

Clinical approach
The first priority is to exclude hyperkalaemia, a life-threatening complication of renal failure (see *Emergency medicine*, Section 1.15 and *Nephrology*, Section 1.6). This is not present in this case, and the house officer is correct in her assessment. One week after surgery the woman clearly had significant renal impairment, which could have been acute (precipitated by the immediate effects of hip fracture or surgery) or chronic, and her drug treatment is very likely to have induced further acute deterioration in renal function.

The background treatment with both laxative and diuretic therapy might have resulted in underfilling of the circulation, when the renin–angiotensin system is activated and glomerular filtration is critically dependent on afferent and efferent glomerular arteriolar tone. The use of non-steroidal anti-inflammatory drugs in this situation is undesirable because blockade of the afferent glomerular arteriolar dilatation (as a result partly of vasodilator prostaglandins) may reduce glomerular filtration further, making dependence on the activated renin–angiotensin system even more critical. Introduction of an ACE inhibitor would be the last straw, because glomerular filtration could not be sustained and renal function inevitably deteriorated.

The episode of 'heart failure' may have been caused by excessive fluid administration in the immediate postoperative period, or may have resulted from pre-existing cardiac disease, further contributing to underperfusion of the kidneys and predisposing to acute-on-chronic renal failure.

The electrolytes and renal function tests should have been much more closely monitored. The patient's clinical deterioration resulted from uraemia exacerbated by the retention of, and increased sensitivity to, the opiate analgesic contained in the compound preparation co-codamol.

Management required removal of the drugs contributing to nephrotoxicity, careful restoration of circulatory volume (with monitoring of central venous pressure) and withdrawal of opioid analgesics. Naloxone could have been administered if the clinical state warranted this.

Table 31 Reduced glomerular function is the primary concern with regards to abnormal drug handling in renal failure. Other mechanisms can contribute to altered drug responses.

Abnormality	Effect	Mechanism
Pharmacokinetic		
Primary importance	Reduced renal clearance	Reduced glomerular filtration
		Reduced tubular secretion
Secondary considerations	Reduced drug absorption	Increased gastric pH
		Binding of drugs to phosphate-binding agents
	Reduced protein binding	Acidosis
		Low serum albumin
	Drug volume of distribution may be altered	
Pharmacodynamic	Increased sensitivity	CNS depressants
		Hypotensives or fluid-retaining drugs according to fluid balance
		Anticoagulants
		Neostigmine (reduced cholinesterase activity)

The kidney is the major site of drug excretion; renal impairment is therefore associated with significant alterations in the pharmacokinetic parameters of many drugs (Table 31). Renal disease may also be associated with altered pharmacodynamic responses that may be:
• enhanced, e.g. increased sensitivity to sedative drugs or antiplatelet agents
• reduced, e.g. reduced sensitivity to diuretics.
Many drugs can exacerbate renal impairment, which is not always reversible.

Problems with toxicity are most likely to occur with drugs that have a narrow therapeutic window and are highly dependent on renal excretion for clearance (e.g. digoxin, aminoglycosides, lithium). The doses of such drugs, which are excreted by the kidney as parent compound or active metabolite, may need to be modified, depending on laboratory estimates of the degree of renal impairment. The plasma concentration of some drugs may be monitored (e.g. digoxin, lithium, aminoglycosides, cyclosporin). Always consider the contribution of dialysis to drug clearance in patients on renal replacement therapy.

Table 32 The creatine clearance can be estimated from the serum creatinine. The severity of renal impairment can then be determined and altered dosing regimens implemented.

Grade	Creatinine clearance (GFR) (mL/min)	Serum creatinine (approx.) (μM)
Mild	20–50	150–300
Moderate	10–20	300–700
Severe	<10	>700

Renal impairment may be divided arbitrarily into three grades for the purposes of prescribing medication (Table 32). These grades correspond to those used by the pharmaceutical industry in the product labelling information provided with all medications.

The Cockroft and Gault formula

Male's creatinine clearance = [1.1 × (150 − Age) × Body weight (kg)]/[72 × Plasma creatinine conc. (μmol)]
Female's creatinine clearance = [0.9 × (150 − Age) × Body weight (kg)]/[72 × Plasma creatinine conc. (μmol)]

Adjustment of drug dosage in renal impairment

The clinical development of new drugs includes studies specifically conducted in patients with impaired renal function to provide data on alterations in pharmacokinetics and pharmacodynamics. The half-life of drugs excreted in an active form by the kidney will be prolonged in renal impairment if the dosage is not modified. The degree of renal impairment that necessitates a dose adjustment will depend on:
• alternative clearance mechanisms available for the drug
• the degree of toxicity of the drug.
An adjustment of the initial or loading dose is not usually necessary because the volume of distribution for the drug is generally similar for the uraemic and the healthy subjects. Subsequent doses should be based on the severity of renal impairment and involve either:
• usual maintenance doses given less frequently or
• a lower maintenance dose given at the same frequency as in the healthy subject.

Furosemide in renal failure

There are two main pathways of tubular secretion that affect weak organic acids and weak organic bases (see Fig. 9). The organic acids that accumulate in renal failure compete with drugs that are normally secreted through this route. One such drug is furosemide (frusemide), which must enter the tubular lumen to act. Much higher doses of furosemide need to be given to patients with renal impairment, partly to overcome the competition from organic acids that block its tubular secretion.

Assessment of the severity of renal impairment

The serum creatinine alone may not accurately predict renal function and the most important parameter is the creatinine clearance, either assessed by the Cockroft and Gault formula or determined directly.

	Mechanism	Example
Pre-renal	Excessive water and electrolyte loss	Diuretics and laxatives
	Increased afferent arteriolar tone	Non-steroidal anti-inflammatory drugs
		Cyclosporin
	Reduced efferent arteriolar tone	ACE inhibitors
	Hypercatabolism	Tetracyclines
Renal	Acute tubular necrosis resulting from direct tubular damage (esp. proximal)	Aminoglycosides
		Vancomycin
		Amphotericin B
		Cefaloridine
		Radiocontrast agents
		Ciclosporin
		Cisplatin (and other anticancer agents)
		Paracetamol overdosage (mechanism as for hepatotoxicity)
	Acute interstitial nephritis	Penicillins
		Non-steroidal anti-inflammatory drugs
		Thiazide diuretics
'Post-renal'	Deposition of drug or metabolite in renal tubule with secondary damage to tubular cells	Sulphonamides
		Cytotoxics due to urate deposition
		Aciclovir
		Methotrexate
	Induction of formation of renal calculi	Vitamin D and calcium supplements

Table 33 Mechanisms by which drugs can cause an acute deterioration in renal function

The time to reach steady-state concentrations is dependent only on the drug half-life. Prolongation of the half-life in renal disease will delay the time taken to reach steady-state concentrations.

Renal function may continue to deteriorate with time and further alterations in the drug regimen may be required. In the face of changing renal function, it is important to monitor patients carefully for signs of drug toxicity, either by using pharmacodynamic outcomes (e.g. blood sugar in patients receiving sulphonylureas, pulse rate in patients receiving atenolol) or, when appropriate, using drug plasma concentration measurements.

When faced with prescribing for a patient with renal impairment:
• First check if a dosage reduction is indicated from a standard reference such as the *British National Formulary* (see Appendix 3).
• The data sheet provided with the drug should indicate appropriate dose alterations according to the severity of renal impairment, or alternatively use a standard reference such as *Avery's Drug Treatment*, Appendix D, Guide to Drug Dosage in Renal Failure.

Nephrotoxic drugs

Many drugs can contribute to an acute (Table 33) or chronic (Table 34) reversible or irreversible deterioration

Table 34 Drugs commonly implicated in contributing to chronic decline in renal function.

Mechanism	Types of agent	Examples
Direct toxicity	Immunosuppressants	Cyclosporin
	Cytotoxics	Cisplatin
	Analgesics	Non-steroidal anti-inflammatory drugs
Indirect toxicity	Cytotoxics	Urate toxicity
	Uricosurics	Urate toxicity
	Vitamin D	Hypercalcaemia

in renal function. The kidneys are particularly susceptible to the toxic effects of drugs because they receive a high cardiac output and have a commensurately high metabolic activity. The kidneys are the final common pathway for the excretion of many drugs and toxic metabolites, and the effects of such toxicity are likely to be more severe in the face of chronic diminished renal reserve.

Nephrotoxic drugs should be avoided if possible in patients with renal disease.

British National Formulary, Appendix 3.
Speight TM, Holford HG, eds. *Avery's Drug Treatment*, 4th edn. ADIS Press.

Drug development and rational prescribing

The processes of development of drugs from identification of molecules to their release as medicines into the marketplace are outlined in this section (Fig. 30).

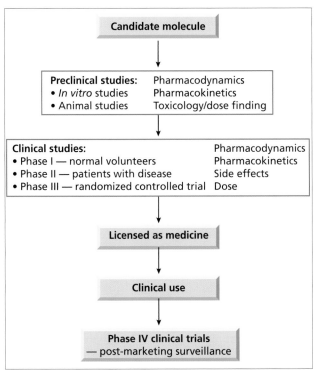

Fig. 30 Drug development—from molecule to market place.

6.1 Drug development

6.1.1 IDENTIFYING MOLECULES FOR DEVELOPMENT AS DRUGS

As an example, we consider the development of new drugs for diabetes.

Identifying new candidate molecules for the treatment of diabetes

Insulin resistance is a common feature of type 2 diabetes and obesity. In the early 1980s, new compounds were sought that could treat these conditions by decreasing insulin resistance. Ciglitazone was selected as a promising candidate because it was shown to reduce insulin resistance in animal models of diabetes. Based on this discovery a range of related chemical compounds, the

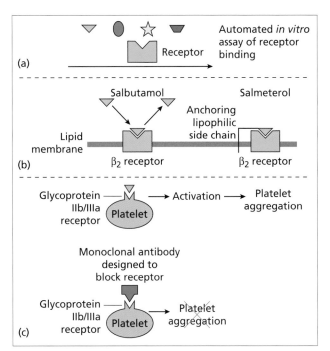

Fig. 31 Identification of molecules for development as drugs. (a) Molecules may be screened for therapeutic effect, e.g. by automated *in vitro* assays of binding to a specific receptor, or by examination of the effect of molecules in animal models of disease. (b) Molecules may be modified from other molecules of known effect, e.g. salbutamol is a short-acting β_2-receptor agonist and salmeterol is a long-acting β_2-receptor agonist, because the addition of a lipophilic side chain allows it to remain anchored in the cell membrane adjacent to the β_2-receptor and slows washout from the receptor. (c) Molecules may be synthesized for a specific therapeutic purpose. Antibodies can be designed to target undesirable proteins or cells in the body, e.g. monoclonal antibodies that bind to the platelet IIb/IIIa glycoprotein receptor inhibit platelet aggregation.

thiazolidinediones or glitazones, was synthesized and tested for antihyperglycaemic activity in diabetic animal models. The more potent of these compounds were selected for development for use in the clinical setting.

 A number of different approaches are used to identify molecules that may have therapeutic use (Fig. 31):
- screening of molecules for therapeutic effect
- modification of identified molecules
- design of molecules for a specific therapeutic purpose.

Preclinical studies of new drugs

Preclinical studies are performed either *in vitro*, e.g. in cell culture systems or tissues, or in animals, before giving the drug to humans. The purpose of preclinical studies is to establish the following:

- What actions the drug has (pharmacodynamics)
- How the drug is absorbed, distributed, metabolized and eliminated (pharmacokinetics)
- What toxic effects the drug has after a single dose, repeated doses and long-term administration (toxicology)
- What doses of the drug are effective but also likely to be safe.

Pharmacodynamics

Early studies with glitazones showed that these compounds suppressed insulin resistance and hyperglycaemia in genetically obese diabetic rats. Subsequent *in vitro* and animal studies revealed that they bind and activate a nuclear receptor, peroxisome proliferator-activated receptor γ (PPARγ). PPARγ activation results in the modulation of transcription of a number of insulin-responsive genes involved in the control of glucose and lipid metabolism.

Pharmacokinetics

In vitro studies of the effect of mice hepatic cytosol and microsome preparations on the glitazones predicted that these drugs would be metabolized by liver enzymes. The interaction between cytochrome P450 enzymes and individual glitazones was also assessed *in vitro*, predicting that troglitazone and its metabolites would inhibit CYP 2C8, 2C9, 2C19 and CYP 3A4 activity, whereas rosiglitazone and pioglitazone would be metabolized by these enzymes but would not inhibit them.

In vivo studies of glitazone pharmacokinetics in dogs and rats were used to establish that the drugs were absorbed across the gastrointestinal tract, widely distributed in tissues, metabolized in the liver, and largely excreted in the bile and faeces, with the remainder being eliminated in the urine.

Toxicology

As the glitazones are likely to be given to patients over a prolonged period, long-term studies looking for carcinogenic effects of glitazones in animals have been performed. Over a 2-year study some rats taking troglitazone developed haemangiosarcomas. The tumour-inducing effects of the glitazones were also found in mouse models of familial adenomatous polyposis and sporadic colon cancer.

Limitations of preclinical studies

Preclinical studies are meant to predict what will happen when the drug is given to humans. These predictions are often difficult because drug effects, metabolism and side effects may differ between conditions *in vitro* and those *in vivo* and between animals and humans. Preclinical

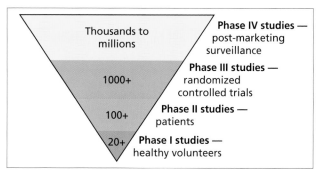

Fig. 32 Numbers of humans exposed to new drugs at different phases of development.

studies to pick up rare or long-term side effects are difficult and expensive to do.

6.1.2 CLINICAL TRIALS: FROM DRUG TO MEDICINE

A drug is any substance that alters physiological processes in the body. A drug can be considered to be a medicine when it is licensed to, and is used to, improve or maintain health. Only a small proportion of drugs that are tested for development become licensed medicines; the lengthy path that they have to follow is shown in Figs 30–32.

Phases of clinical trials

The phases of clinical trials are illustrated in Fig. 32.

Phase I trials

Phase I trials test drug handling by healthy volunteers. They are the first tests done in humans and include:
- Pharmacodynamic studies: some assessment of drug actions in people without disease.
- Assessment of types and risk of side effects.
- Pharmacokinetic studies: absorption, distribution, metabolism and elimination of the drug. Potential drug interactions may also be identified at this stage.
- Dose-finding studies: determination of plasma concentration, effects and side effects at different doses to establish safety and efficacy.

Drugs that are potentially harmful, e.g. chemotherapeutic agents, will not be given to normal volunteers.

Phase II trials

Phase II trials test drug handling and effects in people with disease. They are the first tests done in patients and include the following:
- Pharmacodynamic studies: first assessment of drug efficacy in people with disease.

• Reassessment of types and risk of side effects in patients.
• Reassessment of pharmacokinetics and drug dose in patients.

Phase III trials

Phase III trials formally assess the effectiveness and safety (and acceptability) of the drug in people with disease. The gold standard phase III study is the double-blind, randomized controlled trial (RCT). In the simplest form of RCT, people with the condition expected to respond to a new drug are allocated randomly into two groups. One group receives the active drug and the other placebo. Drug and placebo look identical and neither the investigator nor the trial subjects know who is taking what. Both groups of subjects are monitored for treatment effects and adverse reactions, and statistical methods are used to determine whether beneficial and harmful effects are significantly different in people taking the drug from those seen in people taking placebo. RCTs can also be used to compare the safety and efficacy of a new drug with existing treatment.

Licensing

Before a drug can be used as a medicine in the UK, it has to be granted a licence—known as a marketing authorization. To achieve this licence, the company manufacturing the drug has to collect evidence from preclinical and clinical trials of the drug's efficacy, and must show that the drug meets initial safety requirements for use in the proposed indications. In addition, data about the pharmaceutical quality of the drug preparation must also be demonstrated (Fig. 33).

A product licence gives reassurance about efficacy, safety and pharmaceutical quality. Safety data at the time of product launch are always very limited and the true safety may take years to become apparent (see Fig. 30). Evidence of efficacy does not necessarily mean that a drug is an effective treatment.

Licensing process

Applications for marketing authorization in the UK can be made either to the UK licensing authority or to the European Medicines Evaluation Agency (EMEA) (see Fig. 33). Marketing authorizations, once granted, last for 5 years.

The UK Licensing Authority is made up of four government ministers with responsibility for health. The executive arm of the licensing authority is the Medicines Control Agency (MCA). Applications for marketing authorization for a new product are assessed by the MCA, which takes advice from other bodies, particularly the Committee on Safety of Medicines (COSM), on questions of the safety, quality and efficacy of new medicines for human

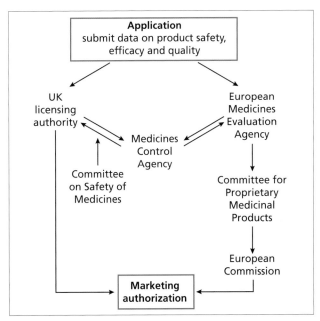

Fig. 33 Licensing mechanisms for new drugs.

use. The assessment procedure is lengthy, not least because the average quantity of data submitted per application is around 170 volumes, each the size of a telephone directory.

Applications for marketing authorizations can also be made to the EMEA, where they are dealt with by the Committee for Proprietary Medicinal Products (CPMP). The CPMP contracts out assessment work to experts in one of the member states of the European Community (e.g. the MCA), considers the completed assessment and then, after hearing any appeal, delivers an opinion. Successful products are granted an EC authorization by the European Commission, which is valid throughout the European Community.

Postmarketing surveillance (phase IV clinical trials)

News report, 1 December 1997: troglitazone withdrawn in UK because of serious hepatic reactions

Approximately 370 000 patients worldwide have been treated with troglitazone for at least 3 months. Worldwide, 130 cases (6 fatal) of hepatic reactions to troglitazone have been reported, including severe hepatocellular damage, hepatic necrosis and hepatic failure. At present these reactions are unpredictable; no clear patient risk factors for the development of hepatic reactions have been identified, and the reactions can occur from 2 weeks to 8 months after starting the drug. Overall it is considered that, based on present information, the risks of troglitazone therapy outweigh the potential benefits. It has therefore been voluntarily withdrawn from the UK as from 1 December 1997 by the companies concerned, who have informed doctors and pharmacists by letter. Any patient who is taking troglitazone should be transferred to an alternative therapy for the treatment of their diabetes.

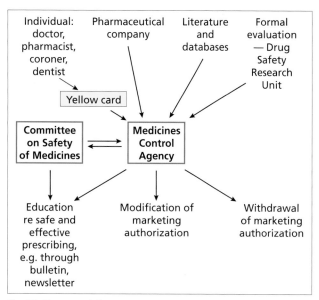

Fig. 34 Pharmacovigilance.

By the time a medicine gets to market it may have been given to only around a thousand people in RCTs (see Fig. 32). These recipients will have been carefully chosen; people at high risk of side effects, such as the very young or old, or those with hepatic or renal impairment will probably have been excluded from the phase III studies. Adverse effects of a drug may not have been identified if they:

- are uncommon
- occur in a vulnerable group of people not included in the clinical trial
- result from unexpected reactions with other drugs, not predicted from trials.

It is important that adverse reactions are detected and acted upon, even after a licence has been granted. Pharmacovigilance is the process of monitoring the use of medicines in everyday practice to detect previously unrecognized adverse reactions (Fig. 34). Pharmacovigilance in the UK is the responsibility of the MCA with the assistance of the CSM.

Adverse reactions to marketed drugs are detected by the following:

- Voluntary reporting: in clinical practice, if an adverse drug reaction is suspected, the professional (doctor, dentist, pharmacist, coroner) voluntarily reports this to the CSM and MCA using the Yellow Card Scheme (see below).
- Compulsory reporting: pharmaceutical companies are under a statutory obligation to report any suspected adverse reactions that come to their attention, e.g. during unpublished clinical trials.
- Literature and database surveillance: reports of adverse reactions in the world literature and from morbidity and mortality databases are documented.
- Formal study: the Drug Safety Research Unit in Southampton carries out formal assessment of selected medicines. The Prescription Pricing Authority is asked to identify all prescriptions of the chosen medicine during a set time period. At the end of this period, questionnaires are sent to the doctors who have written each prescription, asking whether the patient experienced any adverse reaction on the drug. These data give an estimate of the types and frequency of adverse reactions caused by that medicine.

Adverse reactions may be identified, found to be more frequent than expected or shown to affect particular patient subgroups during postmarketing surveillance. These findings may lead to the following:

- Changes in marketing authorization, e.g. restrictions in use or refinement of dose instructions, which allow medicines to be used more safely and effectively.
- Withdrawal of medicines from the market if they are associated with an unacceptable hazard.
- Education of health-care professionals about safer and more effective use of products through modification of product information, newsletters and bulletins.

Practical guide to reporting an adverse drug reaction (ADR)

What should I report?
An ADR is a harmful and unintended effect of a medicine during its use in prevention, treatment or diagnosis of disease. You should report definite or suspected drug reactions (even if not proven) if:
- a product has received its licence or its use has changed in the last 2 years (marked ▼ in the BNF)
- the adverse reaction to ANY product is severe, i.e. 'is fatal, life threatening, disabling, incapacitating or which results in or prolongs hospitalization and/or is medically significant'. *If in doubt—report.*

How do I report an adverse drug reaction?
You fill in a yellow card, which can be found at the back of the BNF. The information required for the report is clearly requested on the card. Even if some of this information is not available, the card should still be sent in. Pharmacists are usually a good source of yellow cards, advice or help if you have problems with this system.

What happens next?
After reporting a suspected ADR, you will receive an acknowledgement letter and a copy of the report to be added to the patient's notes. Cases are then entered on to the MCA's Adverse Drug Reactions On-Line Information Tracking (ADROIT) database. Your information helps the MCA to monitor product safety and take action to minimize risks and maximize benefits of medicines.

Committee on Safety of Medicines: http://www.open.gov.uk/mca/csmhome.htm
Medicines Control Agency: http://www.open.gov.uk/mca/

6.2 Rational prescribing

Entry of new drugs into the market

A medicine receives a licence (marketing authorization) when it has been judged as safe, effective and of sufficient quality by the licensing authority (Fig. 35). A licence, however, does not imply that the drug is better than other drugs also available for the same condition. Once a drug reaches the market, its place in therapy therefore needs to be determined. Ideally this should be done using critical appraisal of the available evidence.

Drugs should be assessed in comparison with other drugs already available for treatment of the same condition on the basis of the following:

- Efficacy: does the new drug work better than existing treatments available for the same condition?
- Safety: does the new drug have fewer or more acceptable side effects than existing treatments?
- Acceptability: is it easier for patients to take this new drug?

If the new drug meets one of these criteria and makes a clinically significant improvement to current therapy then it is likely to be adopted for use.

- Cost: where a new drug does not represent a clinically significant advantage in terms of efficacy, safety or acceptability, it may still be adopted for use if it is as good as, and cheaper than, existing medicines.

Who decides which drugs should be available for prescription?

Decisions are made at the level of the individual, the institution, the health authority and nationally. At each level, the decision-making process is used to develop a list or set of drugs that will be used in clinical practice.

Individuals become familiar with a small number of drugs (usually 50–200) that they are comfortable prescribing. New drugs are added to this list or rejected based on, for example, clinical evidence, anecdotal experience, views of colleagues and marketing pressures.

Institutions may develop a 'formulary' which lists drugs that are acceptable for prescription in that institution. The aim of the formulary is to promote best practice, by allowing prescribing only of drugs that are proven to be safe, effective and acceptable. Formularies are also used to try to reduce drug costs for an institution by encouraging prescribing of the cheapest effective drugs for each condition.

The National Institute for Clinical Excellence (NICE) is a national organization set up by the government. NICE uses standard criteria of efficacy, safety, acceptability and cost to assess medicines, but also takes into account medical, economic, social and 'moral' perspectives when deciding whether or not the drug should be available for prescription on the NHS.

In practice, decisions about drugs that will be available for prescription are made at all levels and there are advantages and disadvantages to each (Table 35).

6.2.1 CLINICAL GOVERNANCE AND RATIONAL PRESCRIBING

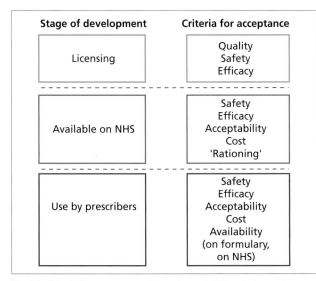

Stage of development	Criteria for acceptance
Licensing	Quality Safety Efficacy
Available on NHS	Safety Efficacy Acceptability Cost 'Rationing'
Use by prescribers	Safety Efficacy Acceptability Cost Availability (on formulary, on NHS)

Fig. 35 Criteria for acceptance of new drugs at different stages of development.

Example 29: A tale of two heart attacks

Patient A
A patient is admitted to hospital with suspected myocardial infarction. Immediately on arrival the diagnosis is confirmed by ECG, and he is given 300 mg of aspirin to chew and thrombolysis is started within 20 minutes of his coming through the door of the A&E department. He is transferred to the coronary care unit (CCU), where he receives a statin, β blockers and an ACE inhibitor, and continues aspirin. These treatments continue on discharge.

Table 35 Decision-making and rational prescribing.

Decision-making level	Advantages	Disadvantages
Individual prescriber	In touch with patients needs If individual makes the decision they are more likely to implement it Process of critical appraisal helps with continued education	Insufficient time available for detailed appraisal required Inefficient if same process is repeated, e.g. by 100 000 doctors Responsibility for, e.g. cost, decisions may interfere with doctor–patient relationship Individual decisions heavily influenced by personal bias
Institution (hospital primary care group)	Decisions relevant to local needs Local ownership of decisions may improve implementation	Inefficient if same work is repeated in many institutions Inequalities where different institutions reach different decisions
Health authority	Decisions made at distance from prescriber–patient relationship Decision less subject to clinician bias (but more subject to manager bias?)	Inefficient if same work is repeated in many regions Variability leads to 'postcode prescribing' Decisions may not take account of local need Decisions divorced from clinical situation therefore less likely to be supported or implemented
Government decision on basis of advice from National Institute for Clinical Excellence (NICE)	Decisions made at national level, removing local and regional variability Government can be blamed for cost decisions, protecting relationship of health-care providers with patients Efficient as work needs to be done only once and disseminated to all prescribers	Out of touch with needs of patients and prescribers Slow and bureaucratic Perceived as a threat to autonomy by doctors Subject to change with political climate Subject to economic pressures, e.g. from pharmaceutical companies which may threaten to withdraw income, jobs, etc.

Example 29: A tale of two heart attacks (*continued*)

Patient B
A patient is admitted to hospital with suspected myocardial infarction. As the admitting department is exceptionally busy, he waits 4 h for the ECG to be done and to be reported by the on-call senior house officer. The doctor who attends the patient has recently seen a patient die from intracerebral haemorrhage after thrombolysis and is reluctant to give this treatment. Eventually, after discussion with colleagues, thrombolysis is started 6 h after the patient arrived in A&E and 12 h after the pain commenced. Aspirin is forgotten in the confusion. The patient is admitted to a medical ward as there are no beds on the CCU. He is not seen during his admission by a senior doctor and is ultimately discharged by the house officer on aspirin and isosorbide mononitrate. (See *Emergency medicine*, Section 1.3, and *Cardiology*, Section 1.5.)

Patient A receives evidence-based, well-organized treatment. Patient B receives poorly organized treatment in which the evidence has largely been forgotten or ignored.
• What factors could have led to inferior treatment for patient B?
• How can we ensure that more patients receive the best treatment available?

Introduction

Clinical governance has become a catch phrase that is used by many but understood by few. It can be encapsulated by a few simple concepts.

It is desirable for every patient to receive the best care available as defined by current evidence.

Many factors, some of which are illustrated by patient B, get in the way of individual patients receiving the best possible care, including the following:
• Practitioners lack knowledge of best available care
• Practitioners have personal bias for or against bad or good practice
• Practitioners are overstretched and therefore forget to, or are unable to, provide best care
• Practitioners may not be motivated to provide best care
• Resources are not available (e.g. beds, drugs, staff, theatre time) to provide best care.

Clinical governance describes a symbiotic relationship between individuals and institutions, which attempts to overcome these factors and enable good medical practice and high standards of care to be achieved. The individual accepts responsibility to work in a way that is compatible with the values and strategic objectives of the organization (e.g. hospital or primary care trust). The organization takes responsibility for the provision of appropriate facilities for medical work and support of professional development of practitioners and clinical teams on a continuing basis.

The process of clinical governance

The process of clinical governance involves the following:
• Setting standards, e.g. by evidence-based guidelines and protocols.

- Monitoring standards, e.g. by clinical audit, risk assessment, patient survey, complaint and critical incident monitoring.
- Maintaining standards through implementation of necessary improvements identified by monitoring, e.g. through staff education, training and development, and through implementation of new research findings.

Clinical governance can make a huge contribution to ensuring that prescribing of medicines in clinical practice is done effectively, safely, acceptably and cost-effectively. Some examples are shown below.

Setting standards

- Formularies can be used to define drugs that are effective, safe, acceptable and cost-effective.
- Best prescribing practice, as assessed by available evidence, can be incorporated into guidelines.
- Guidelines within institutions can include drug doses and methods of administration to reduce prescribing errors.
- National guidelines (NICE) and independent drug reviews (e.g. *Drug and Therapeutics Bulletin, Prescriber's Journal*) can help determine the place of drugs in therapy.

Monitoring standards

- Clinical audit of prescribing practice can ensure that guidelines and formularies are adhered to and that prescribing is cost-effective.
- Monitoring of adverse drug reactions and prescribing errors can be used to assess and limit risk.
- Patient surveys can be performed to determine drug acceptability.

Maintaining standards

- The use of drugs and therapeutics committees can assess new drugs that enter the market.
- A regular update of guidelines should include the place of new drugs in treatment.
- There should be a regular review of older medicines.
- There should be training and education of all practitioners in the principles of rational prescribing and critical appraisal, which might be performed by clinical pharmacologists and clinical pharmacists.

How can clinical governance help?

Clinical governance can help to overcome some of the problems that led to patient B receiving unsatisfactory treatment for his myocardial infarction. In theory the use of many aspects of clinical governance should ensure that:

- patients with chest pain are treated as priority and receive an immediate ECG, which is reported without delay
- patients receive thrombolysis according to need, irrespective of an individual practitioner's bias
- 'door-to-needle time' is minimized to ensure that thrombolysis is given as quickly as possible
- standard treatment guidelines (based on evidence) are followed so that treatment is not forgotten even when busy (aspirin) or when the practitioner is not personally aware of current evidence (discharge medication).

In this case, it was also the responsibility of the individual physician in charge to review the patient regularly and to ensure implementation of good medical practice and the responsibility of the institution, e.g. to provide adequate staff to see urgent patients more quickly and to provide adequate facilities, e.g. CCU beds.

See General clinical issues, Section 4.

6.2.2 RATIONAL PRESCRIBING, IRRATIONAL PATIENTS?

Example 30: Living in the 'real world'

Case history
You review a 55-year-old man in a general medical clinic who has hypertension and type 2 diabetes. He has been prescribed lisinopril 10 mg once daily. His blood pressure is 180/110 mmHg and he has proteinuria. His creatinine is 200 µmol/L. On close questioning, he admits that he has not taken any of the tablets.

- Why might patients not take prescribed medication?
- What are the implications for this patient in not taking antihypertensive medication?
- How might you approach the consultation?

Patients not taking the prescribed medication

As many as 50% of people with chronic illness do not take their medication in optimal doses and so do not derive the optimal benefits of treatment. This is true even where the consequences of not taking treatment may be life threatening. For example, about 22% of recipients of renal transplants miss doses of immunosuppressive medication and 60–70% of patients with HIV omit doses of antiretroviral therapy.

Failure to take prescribed medication and its impact on health

Non-adherence to or non-compliance with treatment has considerable health and economic costs for both individuals and society. Non-adherence to prescribed treatment contributes significantly to premature death from many conditions, including asthma, cardiovascular disease, epilepsy and diabetes. Non-adherence increases morbidity, which increases requirements for health care and results in lost working days and reduced productivity. Non-adherence to antituberculosis medication or antibiotics may lead to spread of infection or emergence of resistant organisms, which endanger other members of society.

Reasons for non-adherence to treatment

There are many reasons why patients do not take prescribed medication. Common reasons include the following:
• Lack of confidence in the efficacy of medicines, or in the advice of doctors
• Perception that medication is unnecessary
• Intolerance of side effects
• Fear of ill effects of medication over time, e.g. addiction or immunity to medicines, development of cancer
• Experiences or advice from relatives or friends regarding the medication
• Stigma attached to taking treatment, e.g. for HIV, TB or mental illness
• Difficulty taking medication in daily routine or forgetting to take medication
• Lack of information about medicines or inability to understand which medicines to take and when.

Impact of the prescribing encounter

The relationship between doctor and patient and the quality of the 'prescribing encounter' can have a substantial impact on the likelihood that the patient will take the prescribed medication. Several different models of medical encounters have been described.

Paternalistic prescribing encounter

The doctor decides what treatment to implement, informs the patient of this choice and its implications, and prescribes the drug. The patient is compliant (or non-compliant) with treatment.

Shared model

The doctor and patient share medical and other relevant information, and participate in all stages of the decision-making process simultaneously. The prescription is the outcome of joint deliberation. The doctor and patient reach agreement (concordance) on the treatment to be tried.

It is expected (but not unequivocally proven) that the shared model would improve adherence to treatment by allowing the patient to discuss beliefs and fears when starting new medication and to have some ownership in the decision to take the drug. Concordance allows that the view of the patient is as important as, if not more important than, the doctor's view in making the prescribing decision. The decision not to take treatment is therefore perfectly valid, providing that it is made in the light of full and accurate information.

Example 30: Living in the 'real world' *(continued)*

Clinical approach
This patient has renal impairment with hypertension and type 2 diabetes mellitus. Control of his blood pressure is essential to slow further deterioration of his renal function, as well as to reduce his risk of vascular disease.

A lecture on the stupidity of not taking tablets is unlikely to make any difference to his adherence to treatment and may deter him from attending for further follow-up. Ideally, discussion in the consultation will explore knowledge, attitudes and beliefs of both doctor and patient, which include:
• the nature and severity of his illness
• reasons for taking or not taking medication
• feasibility of the proposed treatment regimen.
Negotiation around these issues should lead to agreement about a course of action.

BMJ 7212, 19/8/99. Embracing patient partnership
Concordance group website: http://www.concordance.org

7 Self-assessment

Answers are on pp. 98–101.

Question 1
A 45-year-old man is taking long-term theophylline for asthma. One evening, he is admitted to the Accident and Emergency department with convulsions. You suspect theophylline toxicity. Which one of the following statements is true?

A his convulsions should not be treated until a theophylline level is available

B theophylline toxicity may have been precipitated by the concomitant prescription of phenytoin

C theophylline toxicity may have been precipitated by the concomitant prescription of erythromycin

D theophylline toxicity only occurs in the elderly

E theophylline is an example of a drug with a wide therapeutic range (therapeutic index)

Question 2
A 60-year-old woman is admitted feeling generally unwell. Her serum potassium is found to be elevated at 7.0 mmol/l. Which of the following drugs is the LEAST likely to have contributed to her hyperkalaemia?

A lisinopril

B bendrofluazide

C losartan

D spironolactone

E slow-release potassium chloride

Question 3
A 40-year-old woman has developed haemolytic anaemia secondary to drug therapy. Which of the following drugs is NOT a well-recognised cause of haemolytic anaemia?

A phenoxymethylpenicillin

B mefenamic acid

C methyldopa

D ranitidine

E rifampicin

Question 4
A 52-year-old lady who is on some regular medication presents with a sore throat and fever. You check a full blood count and find that the patient has developed neutropenia. Which of the following drugs is most likely to have caused this side effect?

A captopril

B carbimazole

C carvedilol

D ciprofloxacin

E clomipramine

Question 5
A 65-year-old gentleman attending the cardiology clinic complains of swelling and tenderness of his breasts. You diagnose probable gynaecomastia. Which of the following drugs is most likely to be the cause?

A Simvastatin

B Amiodarone

C Digoxin

D Aspirin

E Ramipril

Question 6
A patient presents with acute dystonia and oculogyric crisis after being treated with metoclopramide. Which statement is true with regards to this adverse drug reaction?

A it occurs only after long-term use of metoclopramide

B it is most common in middle-aged men

C it can persist for several days after withdrawal

D it does not occur with prochlorperazine

E it is best treated with procyclidine

Question 7
A patient has developed abnormal thyroid function tests after being started on amiodarone two months ago. Which one of the following features, in conjunction with clinical symptoms and signs, is helpful in diagnosing overt hypothyroidism?

A increase in thyroid-stimulating hormone (TSH) up to 20 mU/L

B decrease in T3

C elevated free T4 and T3

D T4 at upper end of or just above normal range

E low free T4, and low T3

Question 8
A 17-year-old boy fails to breathe spontaneously after an operation. Talking to his family, his sister has previously had similar problems. Which of the following drugs could have caused this problem?

A thiopentone

B atracurium

C suxamethonium

D cisatracurium

E halothane

Question 9

A 58-year-old man with elevated cholesterol has failed to reach a desired cholesterol level on statin treatment. You decide to commence him on ezetimibe. Which of the following is true concerning ezetimibe?

A prescription with statin treatment is contraindicated

B decreased absorption of fat soluble vitamins is an unwanted effect

C its main action is to prevent cholesterol synthesis by the liver

D it causes an elevation in plasma triglyceride concentrations

E it causes a reduction in low-density lipoprotein (LDL)-cholesterol of approximately 20%

Question 10

A 73-year-old man with dementia attends clinic with his wife. She has heard about memantine and wonders if it would be suitable for her husband. Which one of the following is true of memantine?

A it has no interaction with amantadine

B it is licensed for patients with all types of dementia

C it inhibits renal excretion of ranitidine

D it enhances the effects of barbiturates

E it is an acteylcholinesterase inhibitor

Question 11

A 24-year-old Type I diabetic is currently on a basal-bolus regime, comprising twice daily basal isophane insulin complemented by short-acting insulin at meal times. He has recently heard about insulin glargine and wonders if it would be suitable for him. Which statement concerning insulin glargine is true?

A it is formulated by adding zinc suspension to insulin

B it is rapid-acting and should be injected just before meals

C it is particularly useful for patients troubled by hypoglycaemic episodes

D it needs to be mixed thoroughly before injecting

E it has little effect on fasting blood glucose

Question 12

A 72-year-old white woman has uncomplicated essential hypertension. Her blood pressure is 162/102 mmHg despite optimization of non-pharmacological therapy. Which one of the following would you choose as the first-line treatment for her?

A atenolol 50 od

B bendrofluazide 2.5 mg od

C bendrofluazide 5 mg od

D enalapril 5 mg od

E ramipril 2.5 mg od

Question 13

A 48-year-old Afro-Caribbean man has uncomplicated essential hypertension with blood pressure 154/102 mmHg despite optimization of non-pharmacological therapy. Which one of the following would you use as the first-line treatment in this patient?

A atenolol 50 mg od

B nifedipine 10 mg tds

C amlodipine 5 mg od

D ramipril 2.5 mg od

E enalapril 5 mg bd

Question 14

A middle-aged man is brought by ambulance to the Medical Admissions Unit. He was fitting when picked up and is still having a grand mal convulsion. The most appropriate treatment is:

A lorazepam 2 mg intravenously

B fosphenytoin 15 mg/kg body weight phenytoin equivalent, intravenously at a rate of 100–150 mg phenytoin equivalent/min

C phenytoin 15 mg/kg body weight, intravenously at a rate of 50 mg/min

D diazepam 10 mg intravenously

E phenobarbitone 10 mg/kg body weight, intravenously at a rate of 100 mg/min

Question 15

In a healthy volunteer study, the diuretic response to intravenous doses of loop diuretics A, B and C were compared. A 1 mg dose of diuretic A produced a similar diuresis to 40 mg of diuretic B and 50 mcg of diuretic C. It was found that maximal doses of A produced a similar diuresis to maximal doses of B, but the response obtained with maximal doses of C was considerably lower than that of A or B. Which of the following statements is correct in relation to the action of A, B and C:

A drugs A and B are of similar potency

B drug C is more potent than drug A but of lower efficacy

C drug C is of lower potency than drugs A and B but of greater efficacy

D drug A is of greater efficacy than drugs B and C

E no conclusion can be drawn regarding the relative efficacy and potency of the three drugs

Question 16

A 48-year-old woman with a renal transplant is established on ciclosporin, azathioprine and prednisolone to prevent transplant rejection, and enalapril and bendrofluazide for hypertension. After a 14-day course of ketoconazole for oesophageal candidiasis her creatinine is found to have increased from 100 µmol/L to 180 µmol/L. Her deterioration in renal function is most likely attributable to:

A hypertension poorly controlled on enalapril and bendrofluazide

B nephrotoxic effects of ketoconazole

C ciclosporin toxicity due to inhibition of ciclosporin metabolism by ketoconazole

D transplant rejection due to induction of ciclosporin metabolism by ketoconazole

E effect of enalapril on background of stenosis of artery supplying renal transplant

Question 17

Clozapine is an atypical antipsychotic drug that appears to have fewer problems with adverse effects than older antipsychotics. The relative safety of clozapine stems from which one of the following properties:

A low affinity for dopamine D2 receptors

B low affinity for 5HT receptors

C increase in prolactin levels

D does not cause tachycardia

E no effect on white cell counts

Question 18

A 39-year-old woman with a past history of treated hypertension is in her 3rd trimester of pregnancy and requires on-going anti-hypertensive treatment. Which anti-hypertensive would you definitely NOT prescribe?

A hydralazine

B labetalol

C lisinopril

D methyldopa

E nifedipine

Question 19

A 70-year-old woman has severe Parkinson's disease and is on co-careldopa and apomorphine. She complains of nausea and vomiting due to her medication. Which one of the following drugs would you prescribe for these symptoms?

A domperidone

B metoclopramide

C prochlorperazine

D entacapone

E betahistine

Question 20

A 26-year-old woman presents in the 12th week of pregnancy with fever and dysuria. There is no other significant history, but direct questioning reveals a self-limiting rash in the past after taking penicillin. Urine culture reveals a significant growth of Gram negative bacilli. The organism is sensitive to the antibiotics listed below. Which of the following would be the best choice of drug in this situation?

A ciprofloxacin

B gentamicin

C cefaclor

D trimethoprim

E co-amoxiclav

Question 21

You see a woman in late pregnancy who has just been diagnosed with thyrotoxicosis. She is planning to breast-feed her baby after delivery. Which treatment would you recommend for her?

A carbimazole

B blocking dose of carbimazole with added thyroxine

C potassium perchlorate

D propylthiouracil

E Lugol's iodine

Question 22

A 28-year-old man presents following an overdose. Anti-cholinergic syndrome is suspected. Which one of the following is true of this syndrome?

A tricyclic antidepressants are not a cause

B bradycardia is common

C physostigmine is the treatment of choice

D mydriasis occurs

E urinary incontinence is common

Question 23

A 73-year-old man presents to the Accident and Emergency department with drowsiness and confusion. He is noted to be tachycardic and tachypnoeic. He is not cyanosed, and his pulse oximeter reading is 96% on room air. His wife had been admitted with similar symptoms earlier in the week. Which one of the following is most likely?

A paracetamol overdose

B salicylate overdose

C carbon monoxide poisoning

D cerebrovascular accident

E pneumonia

Question 24

A 79-year-old woman presents to the Accident and Emergency department with confusion, headache and tinnitus. She has recently started on an analgesic for back pain and you are worried she may have taken too much. Which of the following would most likely explain her symptoms?

A paracetamol

B aspirin

C diclofenac sodium

D co-codamol

E codeine phosphate

Question 25

A 35-year-woman presents 6 hours after a deliberate overdose of paracetamol. The paracetamol level is above the treatment line. Thirty minutes after starting an infusion of *N*-acetyl cysteine (NAC) she becomes flushed and hypotensive with a blood pressure of 80/55 mmHg. The infusion is stopped immediately and 500 ml IV 0.9% saline administered over 30 minutes. Which of the following is the correct ongoing management?

A IV chlorphenamine maleate and restart NAC infusion at lowest rate once symptoms resolved

B IV chlorpromazine and restart NAC infusion at lowest rate once symptoms resolved

C IV chlorphenamine maleate and give 2.5 g of oral methionine

D IV chlorpromazine and give 2.5 g of oral methionine

E withhold treatment and recheck paracetamol level at 12 hours

Question 26

A 50-year-old woman has increasing frequency of migraine attacks. You decide to start some prophylactic therapy. Which one of the following drugs would NOT be appropriate for prophylaxis against migraine

A rizatriptan

B sodium valproate

C propranolol

D amitriptyline

E pizotifen

Question 27

A 29-year-old man with a history of epilepsy has been well controlled on carbamazepine and clonazepam for the last 5 years. He now wishes to consider withdrawing from or reducing his medication. Which of the following statements are correct?

A there is about a 60% chance of experiencing a relapse in the first year during withdrawing from anti-epilepsy treatment

B both anti-epileptics can be safely withdrawn simultaneously

C the dose of carbamazepine can be reduced safely by 10% every 2–4 weeks

D he can be advised that he can continue driving during withdrawal from anti-epilepsy treatment as long as she remains free from seizures

E it is likely that he will subsequently require higher doses to regain control with the current therapy, if discontinuation fails

Question 28

You are treating a 72-year-old man with moderate peripheral vascular disease. He exercises regularly but finds that his walking distance is diminishing due to pain. Which drug might help improve pain-free walking distance?

A naftidrofuryl

B cinnarizine

C inositol nicotinate

D simvastatin

E diltiazem

Question 29

A 21-year-old university student complains of difficulty sleeping. She is in the middle of sitting her final exams and would like some medication for a few days to help her sleep. However, she is concerned about potential 'hang-over' effects and would prefer a drug which doesn't cause daytime drowsiness. Which agent would you prescribe?

A diazepam

B midazolam

C promethazine

D loprazolam

E clomethiazole

Question 30

A 74-year-old woman presents with breathlessness. She is a small woman (55 kg) with a chest infection. She is not very unwell, but is in atrial fibrillation at a rate of 170/min. Her electrolytes are normal (K 4.2 mmol/l). As well as treating her pneumonia, you decide to digitalize by prescribing digoxin:

A 0.25 mg orally once daily

B 1.0 mg orally over 24 hours in divided doses

C 1.0 mg intravenously over 20 min

D 0.125 mg orally once daily

E 0.25 mg orally three times daily for one week, then twice daily for one week, then once daily thereafter

Answers to Self-assessment

Statistics, epidemiology, clinical trials, meta-analyses and evidence-based medicine

Answer to Question 1

A

Forest plots are most commonly used in meta-analyses as a concise and elegant way of presenting information from many individual trials, allowing a convenient visual comparison of the separate trial results together with a synthesis of the data.

The horizontal lines emerging from the squares represent confidence intervals. Larger studies have narrower confidence intervals, hence the largest squares are typically associated with the smallest horizontal lines.

Answer to Question 2

B

Most trials evaluate just one treatment. This does not have to be so: factorial trials test two or more treatments simultaneously.

A famous example of a factorial trial was the ISIS-2 study in which comparison was made between placebo and each of two drugs, streptokinase and aspirin. Patients with suspected myocardial infarction were randomised to receive IV streptokinase alone, aspirin alone, both active drugs, or double placebo. The trial showed that each of the drugs produced about a 25% reduction in mortality, also that their effects were additive.

Answer to Question 3

A

Interpreting the sensitivity and specificity of a test depends on what you are using it for.

The poor specificity of this test means that it would be inappropriate to use it as reason for telling people they have HIV infection; in the at-risk population over 50% diagnosed positive will not have the disease. By contrast, the balance of risk is different in screening blood for HIV, where the risk of missing a positive case far outweighs the risk of discarding some blood units unnecessarily, and similarly in looking for bowel cancer.

The test would also potentially be appropriate in screening for head lice where the disease is not serious but you do not want to miss cases and the treatment is simple and safe.

Predictive value depends as much on prevalence of a condition as the sensitivity. The positive predictive value in young patients means most army recruits with a positive test would be false-positive, with more being false-positive than true-positive, but since very few are likely to have heart disease a preliminary screening test with a positive predictive value of 48% would be a reasonable test to use.

Answer to Question 4

D

With a cohort study you start with two (or more) groups with different exposures. This could be exposure to an occupational hazard, or to different drugs or different infections. You then follow them over time to see whether, and when, they develop an outcome (in medicine usually a disease, complication or death). Cohort studies are therefore very good for investigating the effects of rare exposures, as you set the exposure. If the outcome is rare it is unlikely enough cases will occur in the follow-up time to draw any conclusions, so they are not good for rare outcomes.

Unlike other study designs cohort studies follow individuals over time, so are particularly good for measuring incidence of a disease. They are not the best study design for measuring prevalence of a disease in a population (cross-sectional studies are very well designed for this).

Answer to Question 5

E

It is only ethical to conduct a clinical trial if it is capable of detecting a meaningful difference between two treatments to guide future practice. If a trial is underpowered it cannot detect a statistically significant difference. It is therefore mandatory to do a proper power calculation before exposing patients to a clinical trial.

The rather daunting formal definition of a type I error means that a study falsely (but not deliberately) appears to find a difference between two groups which has actually arisen by chance alone. The conventional cut-off of $p < 0.05$ will arise by chance alone one time in twenty. As many thousands of studies are published every month, type I errors are not rare.

A type II error is formally where the null hypothesis is falsely accepted. To claim two treatments are 'equivalent' requires huge numbers, and most studies are underpowered (too small) to reliably rule out a small difference between one treatment and another.

Most published studies are small enough that type I and type II errors are a real possibility, and examples are published in good journals every week.

Answer to Question 6

D

The principle of a crossover design is that a patient has one drug or treatment, then a washout period, and then another drug, and the effect is compared between the two in a single individual. For this reason it is a good study design for treatment of chronic conditions, but not appropriate for acute conditions.

It is just as easy (or difficult) to randomize and double-blind as for other study designs.

Because each person is acting as their own control, it is usually possible to use smaller numbers to get the same power.

Answer to Question 7

B

Case-control studies compare exposures of interest in cases and controls. Two of their great strengths is that they can be used with rare diseases (because cases are pre-selected), and can examine multiple risk-factors (exposures).

They are not good at identifying rare exposures. If the question is whether or not a rare exposure causes a disease then the appropriate design is a cohort study, where one group with the particular exposure of interest is compared with a control group without that exposure.

The greatest difficulty in designing case-control studies is selection of an appropriate control group, and poor control selection often makes otherwise well-conducted studies uninterpretable.

Answer to Question 8

B

Looking at a set of data plotted out on a graph is a good way of determining whether or not it is skewed. There is no such thing as a 'skew test'.

There are few absolutes in statistics, but one is that skewed data should never be described by the mean, as it will lead to misleading distortions.

Chi-squared is for categorical data.

It is possible to use Wilcoxon rank-sum to test the difference between two sets of normally distributed data. However, the Student t-test is more powerful, and so should be used in preference where the data are normally distributed. The rank-sum test is reserved for skewed data, where the t-test cannot be used.

There is no relationship between standard deviation and interquartile range. Interquartile range is a good way of summarising skewed data where the standard deviation (based on the mean) is not appropriate.

Answer to Question 9

E

The first step of EBM involves converting the need for information into an answerable question. To be answerable a question must be focused and should include each of the following four elements:

• A patient or a problem, defined by specific characteristics that are likely to influence the applicability of the evidence

• An intervention: this might be a diagnostic test, a therapeutic intervention, or information concerning prognosis

• A comparison: in questions about diagnosis this might

be with a well-established test; for treatment, it might be with placebo or an alternative treatment

• Outcome measures: it is vital to identify outcome measures that are clinically important, rather than those that are easily measured, e.g. angina, re-infarction and death are more important than thallium scan measurements.

EBM requires explicit use of the best available evidence and its applicability is not restricted to those areas where there is randomised controlled trial evidence.

Answer to Question 10

A

Bias means a flaw in study design that leads to a built-in likelihood that the wrong result may be obtained. It cannot be controlled for at the analysis stage. It can be extremely difficult to design studies without potential bias, particularly when there are complex interactions between exposures under study. Techniques such as restriction and stratification are commonly used to reduce potential for bias.

Answer to Question 11

E

Geographical studies, also called ecological studies, are good at generating hypotheses, but not very helpful in testing them.

Cross-sectional studies, also called prevalence studies, look at the number of cases of a disease at a particular point in time. They are not useful for investigating rare diseases or exposures.

In cohort studies, one group with an exposure of interest is selected and compared over time with another cohort without that exposure. If the control group is well selected, then cohort studies are good for examining the effects of rare exposures, but they are not suited to investigating the cause(s) of a rare disease.

An intervention study cannot be used to look for the cause(s) of a disease.

Answer to Question 12

D

The 95% confidence intervals (95% CI) around a value are the range within which there is a 95% chance that the true value lies. Similarly, the 95% CIs around a difference are the range in which there is a 95% chance that the true difference lies.

If the means of two groups have overlapping 95% CIs, then the two groups are not statistically significantly different. If the 95% CI of the difference between two groups overlaps zero, then the difference between the two groups is not statistically significant.

Statistical and clinical significance should not be confused. A very large study can generate very narrow 95% CIs (or very small p values) for very small differences, which may be of no clinical significance at all. By contrast, a small study may fail to show a statistically significant effect even if the effect is both large and clinically important.

Answer to Question 13
C

Categorical variables are not continuous, e.g. drug/placebo, dead/alive. They should be described as percentages or proportions and compared with a chi-squared test.

Normally distributed continuous data should be described as mean and standard deviation and compared with a Student's *t*-test.

Skewed continuous data should be described as median and range and compared using a test such as the Wilcoxon rank-sum test or the Mann-Whitney U-test.

Answer to Question 14
E

The null hypothesis is always that there is no difference between groups under study.

A type 1 error occurs when 'the null hypothesis is falsely rejected'. In practice this means that the study claims to find a difference that does not really exist, i.e. the result is just a statistical fluke.

A type 2 error occurs when 'the null hypothesis is falsely accepted'. This means that it is claimed that there is no difference between two groups, when in reality the study is simply too small to detect a difference. This type of error can be avoided by making explicit power calculations before embarking on any study. This will answer the question 'if I am studying an outcome that occurs in (say) 20% of a conventionally treated group and want to show a (say) halving in the rate of this outcome, then how many patients do I need to study?'

Answer to Question 15
D

In this study aspirin reduces the risk of DVT/PE from 2.5% to 1.5%: this is an absolute risk reduction of 1% and a proportional (or relative) risk reduction of 1/2.5 = 40%. The NNT to prevent one DVT/PE is 1/absolute risk reduction = 1/0.01 = 100.

Answer to Question 16
C

Whether or not a clinical trial is ethical is governed by the 'uncertainty principle', the fundamental criterion being that both patient and doctor should be substantially uncertain about the appropriateness of each of the trial treatments for that particular patient. If there are strong preferences for one treatment or another (by either the patient or the doctor), then that patient is ineligible: but if both parties are substantially uncertain, then randomisation is appropriate.

Answer to Question 17
B

Skewed data should always be summarized using the median and range. Standard deviation is based on the mean, which is not appropriate for skewed data.

How do you decide if data are skewed? Plot them out and look at them, or find the median and calculate the mean: if these are more than slightly different, then the data is skewed.

Answer to Question 18
A

The clinical significance of a reported reduction in absolute risk, relative risk or odds ratio is not always obvious. The concept of the number needed to treat (NNT) was devised to make this clearer.

If 9.4% of patients given aspirin after myocardial infarction die, compared with 11.8% of those not given aspirin, then the absolute risk reduction produced by aspirin is 11.8 − 9.4 = 2.4%, the relative risk reduction when taking aspirin is 9.4/11.8 = 0.8 (80%), and the NNT is 1 divided by 0.024 = 42, meaning that 42 patients with myocardial infarction must be treated with aspirin to prevent one death.

Answer to Question 19
E

Absolute risk reduction (or increase) = (Risk in group 1) minus (Risk in group 2), which is 2% in this example.

Relative risk is the difference of outcome in one group compared to another = (Risk in group 1) divided by (Risk in group 2). In this case aspirin reduced relative risk by 20%.

The Number Needed to Treat = 1 divided by (Absolute Risk Reduction), which is 1/0.02 or 50 in this example.

Answer to Question 20
D

Chi-squared tests (and variants thereof) are widely used to compare percentages or proportions of categorical data. From the chi-squared statistic a p value is read off a statistical table to give the degree of significance. Traditionally a p value of less than 0.05, indicating a less than 5% probability that a result has arisen by chance, is taken (arbitrarily) as indicating that chance alone is not responsible for the difference between groups.

Normally distributed data can be compared with a Student's *t*-test (with correction for multiple comparisons when appropriate). Skewed continuous data can be compared with a Wilcoxon rank-sum test or a Mann-Whitney U-test.

Clinical pharmacology

Answer to Question 1
C

Convulsions should be treated immediately in the usual way, without waiting for confirmation of the theophylline level.

Theophylline is metabolised by the CYP450 enzymes in the liver. Erythromycin inhibits CYP450 enzymes and increases the half-life of theophylline and hence plasma theophylline concentrations, which may lead to toxicity. By contrast, phenytoin induces CYP450 enzymes, which will decrease the half-life of theophylline and may lead to inadequate therapeutic levels.

Theophylline toxicity is more likely in the elderly due to age-related reduction in the rate of its metabolism, but it can occur at any age.

Theophylline is an example of a drug with a NARROW therapeutic range. It is recommended that plasma theophylline levels be maintained between 10 and 20 mg/l.

Answer to Question 2
B

Bendrofluazide tends to cause hypokalaemia.

The other drugs listed may cause hyperkalaemia, although this is not usually clinically significant when used alone at therapeutic doses. The development of significant drug-induced hyperkalaemia is more likely when more than one of these agents is used in combination, or if the patient has co-existing renal impairment.

Answer to Question 3
D

Drugs can cause haemolytic anaemia by a variety of mechanisms. Penicillin binds covalently to the red blood cell membranes; rifampicin causes immune complex association with red blood cell membranes leading to complement activation; methyldopa and mefenamic acid may induce the formation of autoantibodies against components of red blood cells. Ranitidine is not reported to cause haemolytic anaemia.

Answer to Question 4
B

The anti-thyroid drug carbimazole causes neutropenia in 1 in 800 patients. The Committee of Safety of Medicines (CSM) advise that patients taking carbimazole should be asked to report any symptoms or signs suggestive of infection immediately, especially sore throat. A white blood count should be performed if there is any clinical suspicion of infection, and if there is clinical or laboratory evidence of neutropenia the carbimazole should be stopped promptly.

Answer to Question 5
C

Digoxin is the most likely cause of his gynaecomastia. This side effect is more common with longer-term use and may be unilateral or bilateral. Important differential diagnoses to consider include male breast cancer, liver disease, testicular tumours and hyperthyroidism.

Other drugs that can cause gynaecomastia include oestrogens, spironolactone, cimetidine, verapamil and nifedipine. The gynaecomastia usually improves on stopping the drug or reducing the dose.

Answer to Question 6
E

Dystonic reactions are well-recognized with dopamine receptor antagonists.

They occur shortly after starting therapy, particularly in girls and young women as well as the elderly. The problem usually subsides within 24 hours following cessation of treatment and can be treated with procyclidine 5–10 mg IM (an antimuscarinic).

Answer to Question 7
E

Amiodarone is an iodine rich molecule that resembles T4. A daily dose of 200 mg generates 7 mg free iodine, compared with the WHO optimal intake of 0.15–0.3 mg/day.

This high iodine load blocks further iodide uptake and hormone synthesis by the thyroid, and it also blocks conversion of T4 to T3 and affects the pituitary thyroid axis. The following changes in thyroid function tests can occur within 3 months of starting amiodarone and are not indicative of thyroid disease: increase in TSH up to 20 mU/L, increase in T4 to upper limit of normal range, and decreased T3 levels. The diagnosis of hypothyrodism should be based on clinical assessment, together with the following features: high TSH of > 20 mU/l, low free T4, low T3. Treatment is with thyroxine, aiming for free T4 levels close to the upper limit of the normal range.

Answer to Question 8
C

Suxamethonium is a depolarising neuromuscular blocking agent that is metabolised by plasma pseudocholinesterases. Approximately 1/2500 individuals have deficiency of this enzyme, resulting in prolonged neuromuscular blockade if suxamethonium is given. Management is by prolonged ventilation until the action of the drug wears off. Relatives of affected patients should be screened.

Answer to Question 9

E

Ezetimibe is the first of a novel class of drugs for the treatment of hyperlipidaemia whose main action is to specifically prevent cholesterol absorption from the small intestine. It typically reduces LDL-cholesterol by about 20%, triglycerides by up to 5% and raises HDL-cholesterol by approximately 5%. It does not inhibit the absorption of fat-soluble vitamins, unlike the anion-exchange resins (e.g. colestyramine). Ezetimibe can be safely co-administered with statins and is currently licensed for use in combination with a statin in patients who fail to reach desired lipid profiles or as monotherapy in patients intolerant of a statin. There is no increased risk of myopathy with ezetimibe prescription.

Answer to Question 10

C

Memantine is the first licensed NMDA receptor antagonist for the management of moderate to severe Alzheimer's disease. It has small benefit in reducing deterioration in patients with this condition, but little evidence for use in other types of dementia. Several drug interactions are known:
• NMDA antagonists (e.g. ketamine, amantadine) – can precipitate psychosis
• Dopamine agonists – effects enhanced
• Barbiturates and neuroleptics – effects reduced
• Drugs excreted by cationic transporters in the kidney (e.g. ranitidine, quinine, nicotine) – excretion reduced leading to higher plasma concentrations.

Answer to Question 11

C

Insulin glargine is a long-acting insulin analogue, produced by modifying the chemical structure of insulin. This gives it a smooth, prolonged absorption profile with no peaks. As such, it is a long-acting agent, suitable for providing a basal level of insulin that attempts to mimic the normal physiological state. Its smooth profile reduces the risk of hypoglycaemia, and when given at night it provides good control of the fasting blood glucose. Unlike crystalline suspensions, insulin glargine does not need to be mixed thoroughly prior to injection, making it easier to use.

Answer to Question 12

B

Low-dose diuretics are accepted as the first-line treatment for hypertension in the elderly and appear to confer greater benefit than beta-adrenergic receptor antagonists in this population. Treatment of isolated systolic hypertension in the elderly with the long-acting calcium channel blocker nitrendipine has been shown to reduce stroke and adverse cardiovascular outcome. Calcium channel

blockers may therefore be suitable when diurectics are not tolerated, ineffective or contra-indicated.

Answer to Question 13

C

Calcium-channel blockers (CCBs) and diuretics appear to be the most effective antihypertensives in Afro-Caribbeans. Diuretics have the disadvantage that they commonly cause impotence. Short-acting CCBs do not provide prolonged blood pressure control, can cause reflex tachycardia, and may be associated with higher mortality. A long-acting CCB should be the first-line drug of choice, ideally a once-daily agent that provides smooth 24-hour BP control, e.g. Nifedipine LA 30 mg od or Amlodipine 5 mg od.

ACE (angiotensin-converting enzyme) inhibitors and beta-receptor antagonists are less effective in Afro-Caribbeans, probably because the renin-angiotensin-aldosterone system is usually suppressed in this ethnic group such that drugs that act by suppressing the RAA system are unlikely to be effective.

Answer to Question 14

A

All of these are recognized treatments for status epilepticus. First-line treatment should be with intravenous benzodiazepine, with lorazepam preferred to diazepam because of its longer duration of action. Fosphenytoin is the preferred second-line treatment (phenytoin if this is not available). Phenobarbitone is one of several agents that can be used as third-line treatment, but seek specialist advice if first and second-line treatments are ineffective.

Answer to Question 15

B

The potency of a drug relates to the amount of drug needed to produce a given effect. An equivalent diuresis to that seen with drugs A and B is produced with a considerably smaller dose of C, which is therefore more potent.

Efficacy relates to the maximal response that can be produced by the drug when taken at high dose. Despite increasing the dose, drug C is unable to produce an equivalent maximal diuresis to that obtained with drugs A or B, it is thus of lower efficacy.

The potency of a drug is not often of importance but can become significant if the drug has low solubility and has to be packaged or delivered in such a way that space is limited. Examples might include metered dose aerosols or depot injections.

Answer to Question 16

C

Ketoconazole inhibits liver enzymes that metabolise ciclosporin, increasing plasma ciclosporin concentration and potentially leading to nephrotoxicity. Deterioration in renal function could be seen if enalapril is started on a background of renal artery stenosis, but in this case the close relationship between the timing of the course of ketoconazole and the increase in creatinine makes option C the most likely.

Answer to Question 17

A

Clozapine has fewer extrapyramidal adverse effects than older antipsychotics, which is attributed to its relatively low affinity for D2 dopamine receptors. Unlike older antipsychotics, clozapine has relatively high affinity for 5HT receptors and also has little effect on prolactin levels.

Myocarditis and cardiomyopathy have been reported with atypical antipsychotics, with persistent tachycardia an early warning sign. Agranulocytosis is a well-recognized complication of clozapine: patients should be supervised under the Clozaril Patient Monitoring Service.

Answer to Question 18

C

Evidence underpinning the choice of anti-hypertensive therapy in pregnancy is inadequate to make firm recommendations. There are no reports of serious effects with methyldopa following long and extensive use. Calcium antagonists, labetalol and hydralazine are commonly used, particularly for resistant hypertension in the third trimester. However, angiotensin-converting enzyme (ACE)-inhibitors should be avoided because they may cause oligohydramnios, renal failure and intra-uterine death.

Answer to Question 19

A

Drugs such as apomorphine and bromocriptine cause vomiting through peripheral stimulation of the chemoreceptor trigger zone. Worsening of Parkinson's disease may result from the use of dopamine antagonists, but domperidone is not likely to cross the blood–brain barrier and is therefore the preferred agent in this case. Entacapone is a catechol-O-methyltransferase (COMT) inhibitor that increases levodopa levels, thus worsening nausea and vomiting. Betahistine is used in vertigo.

Answer to Question 20

C

Ciprofloxacin has been associated with arthropathy and cartilage erosions in young animals. Gentamicin needs to be given parenterally and is not suitable for outpatient use, and there is also a risk of fetal nephrotoxicity and ototoxicity. Trimethoprim is a folate antagonist and can

increases the risk of neural tube defects. Co-amoxiclav is a combination of amoxycillin and clavulanic acid, and although there is no definite risk of teratogenicity it should not be used unless absolutely necessary. Furthermore, this patient has previously had a rash with penicillin. Although there is a small risk of cross-allergy (10%) with cephalosporins, cefaclor would be the best choice given that the penicillin allergy was relatively mild and not a full-blown anaphylactic reaction.

Answer to Question 21

D

Anti-thyroid drugs can cross the placenta and breast milk, thus causing hypothyroidism in the child. The carbimazole block-and-replace regimen is the worst in this respect, as the carbimazole crosses the placenta but the thyroxine does not. Potassium perchlorate is no longer used in the UK; Lugol's iodine may occasionally be prescribed for patients undergoing thyroid surgery, but causes goitre in infants. Propythiouracil is more highly protein bound and is ionized at pH 7.4, thus making it less likely to cross the placenta or breast milk.

Answer to Question 22

D

Anticholinergic syndrome occurs following overdose with drugs that have prominent anticholinergic activity, including tricyclic antidepressants, antihistamines and atropine. Features include dry, warm, flushed skin, urinary retention, tachycardia, mydriasis (dilated pupils) and agitation. Although physostigmine, a reversible inhibitor of acteylcholinesterase, is effective in treating symptoms, there is a significant risk of cardiac toxicity (bradycardia, AV conduction defects and asystole). Treatment therefore consists of withdrawal of the precipitating drug and supportive care.

Answer to Question 23

C

This man has carbon monoxide (CO) poisoning. Pulse oximeters cannot distinguish between COHb and HbO_2, therefore it is essential to take arterial blood gases and – to make the specific diagnosis – measure the level of CO. It is important to think about prevention: CO alarms are cheap and readily available.

Answer to Question 24

B

Aspirin in excess causes symptoms of nausea, vomiting, headache, confusion and tinnitus or hearing difficulties. Whilst the co-codamol and codeine phosphate could cause confusion, they would not cause the tinnitus. All analgesics taken for a prolonged period of time can lead to an analgesic-induced headache.

Answer to Question 25
A

Reactions to NAC are well recognized and are not related to hypersensitivity. NAC can almost always be safely restarted and the full treatment dose safely administered after symptomatic treatment. Oral methionine may be an alternative but is definitely second line. IV chlorpromazine would make hypotension worse. Withholding treatment and waiting more than 12 hours would expose the patient to risk of liver failure.

Answer to Question 26
A

Rizatriptan is not used as prophylaxis against migraine. It is a 5HT1 agonist and may be useful in the treatment of acute attacks, for which it is available as either tablets or 'melt wafers' that dissolve on the tongue.

Propranolol and pizotifen are licensed for use as prophylaxis against migraine. Pizotifen may cause drowsiness and weight gain. Sodium valproate and amitriptyline are unlicensed for migraine prophylaxis but can be effective in some patients.

Answer to Question 27
C

About 25% of patients who stop their anti-epilepsy treatment will relapse within a year of starting to taper down their medication. The likelihood of seizure is greatest during withdrawal and in the subsequent 6 months. The DVLA recommends that patients should not drive during this period.

Doses of drugs such as carbamazepine, lamotrigine, phenytoin, sodium valproate and vigabatrin should be reduced by about 10% every 2–4 weeks. Barbiturates, benzodiazepines and ethosuximide should be tapered more slowly by reducing dosage by about 10% every 4–8 weeks. Only one drug should be withdrawn at a time, with a period of 1 month between completing withdrawal of one drug and beginning withdrawal of the next. There

is no evidence to support the belief that patients become resistant to their original therapy following discontinuation.

Answer to Question 28
A

Vasoactive drugs have limited benefit in treating intermittent claudication. There is modest evidence for the use of drugs such as naftidrofuryl and pentoxifylline, but little benefit from cinnarizine or inositol nicotinate. Simvastatin may be prescribed for patients with peripheral vascular disease who have elevated cholesterol levels, but there is no data on improvements in walking distance.

Answer to Question 29
D

Diazepam has a long half-life, principally because of its active metabolites. Midazolam is short-acting but is only used intravenously. Promethazine is an antihistamine with a 12-hour half-life and may cause daytime sedation. Clomethiazole is less safe in overdose, has dependence potential and is only licensed for sedation in the elderly. Loprazolam is short-acting (half-life 6–12 hours) and would be a reasonable choice in this case.

Answer to Question 30
B

The options for treatment of atrial fibrillation are:
• DC cardioversion if the patient is compromised haemodynamically or has ischaemic cardiac pain
• Digoxin – 1.0–1.5 mg orally in divided doses over 24 hours, but can be given intavenously in emergency (0.25-0.5 mg over 10–20 min, repeated after four to eight hours to total intravenous loading dose of 0.5–1.0 mg)
• 'Medical cardioversion' with amiodarone or flecainide
In this clinical context it is likely that the atrial fibrillation (if new) will revert to sinus rhythm as the woman recovers from her pneumonia and most physicians would digitalize in preference to the other options described.

The Medical Masterclass series

Clinical Skills

General Clinical Issues

Pain Relief and Palliative Care

Medicine for the Elderly

Emergency Medicine

Infectious Diseases and Dermatology

Infectious Diseases

Dermatology

Haematology and Oncology

Haematology

Oncology

Cardiology and Respiratory Medicine

Cardiology

2.2.3 Oesophageal tumours
2.2.4 Achalasia
2.2.5 Diffuse oesophageal spasm
2.3 Gastric and duodenal disease
    2.3.1 Peptic ulceration and *Helicobacter pylori*
    2.3.2 Gastric carcinoma
    2.3.3 Rare gastric tumours
    2.3.4 Rare causes of gastrointestinal haemorrhage
2.4 Pancreas
    2.4.1 Acute pancreatitis
    2.4.2 Chronic pancreatitis
    2.4.3 Pancreatic cancer
    2.4.4 Neuroendocrine tumours
2.5 Biliary tree
    2.5.1 Choledocholithiasis
    2.5.2 Cholangiocarcinoma
    2.5.3 Primary sclerosing cholangitis
    2.5.4 Primary biliary cirrhosis
    2.5.5 Intrahepatic cholestasis
2.6 Small bowel
    2.6.1 Coeliac
    2.6.2 Bacterial overgrowth
    2.6.4 Other causes of malabsorption
2.7 Large bowel
    2.7.1 Adenomatous polyps of the colon
    2.7.2 Colorectal carcinoma
    2.7.3 Diverticular disease
    2.7.4 Intestinal ischaemia
    2.7.5 Anorectal disease
2.8 Irritable bowel
2.9 Acute liver disease
    2.9.1 Hepatitis A
    2.9.2 Hepatitis B
    2.9.3 Other viral hepatitis
    2.9.4 Alcohol and alcoholic hepatitis
    2.9.5 Acute liver failure
2.10 Chronic liver disease
2.11 Focal liver lesions
2.12 Drugs and the liver
    2.12.1 Hepatic drug toxicity
    2.12.2 Drugs and chronic liver disease
2.13 Gastrointestinal infections
    2.13.1 Campylobacter
    2.13.2 Salmonella
    2.13.3 Shigella
    2.13.4 Clostridium difficile
    2.13.5 Giardia lamblia
    2.13.6 Yersinia enterocolitica
    2.13.7 Escherichia coli
    2.13.8 Entamoeba histolytica
    2.13.9 Traveller's diarrhoea
    2.13.10 Human immunodeficiency virus (HIV)
2.14 Nutrition
    2.14.1 Defining nutrition
    2.14.2 Protein-calorie malnutrition
    2.14.3 Obesity
    2.14.4 Enteral and parenteral nutrition
    2.14.5 Diets
2.15 Liver transplantation

2.16 Screening, case finding and surveillance
    2.16.1 Surveillance
    2.16.2 Case finding
    2.16.3 Population screening
3 Investigations and practical procedures
3.1 General investigations
3.2 Rigid sigmoidoscopy and rectal biopsy
3.3 Paracentesis
3.4 Liver biopsy

Neurology, Ophthalmology and Psychiatry

Neurology

Nephrology

Rheumatology and Clinical Immunology

Index